Intermittent Fasting

The Code of Weight Loss Mastery in 2019 for Beginners and Advanced. Eat and Stop Obesity.

By Jason Stephens

Table of Contents

hardships that may result from any of the information discussed herein.

Additionally, the information in the following pages is intended only for informational purposes and should thus be thought of as universal. As befitting its nature, it is presented without assurance regarding its prolonged validity or interim quality. Trademarks that are mentioned are done without written consent and can in no way be considered an endorsement from the trademark holder.

Introduction

Congratulations on downloading *Intermittent Fasting* and thank you for doing so. Fasting is a tool that has been used for centuries. From spiritual guides to health experts, it is a practice that has deep roots in our history. You've probably heard a lot and are curious to know if it can help you. With this book, you'll find out not just how it can help, but how much it can help. Intermittent Fasting is one of the best weight loss and management tools around, and this book will be your guide to learning everything you can about it!

The following chapters will discuss topics such as how diets work, and the differences between dieting and fasting. We will also cover some other types of diets, and how Intermittent Fasting differs from them! You will learn how important fasting can be as a tool for good health and gain an in-depth understanding of the effects fasting will have on your body. Is it safe? Is fasting right for you? You're going to find out. With great tips that will make fasting super easy for you, and even a step by step meal plan! And by the end of this quick read, you'll have a firm grasp on Intermittent Fasting and all that goes along with it.

Books similar about the subject floods the market and we thank you again for choosing this one! All efforts were made to make sure useful information was compiled in the book.

Chapter 1: Dieting and How Your Body Responds

With just about a dozen methods of losing weight out on the market, it can be difficult to know what tactic is right for you. We all want to cut those calories down, or maybe we want to just burn them faster. Yet the answers aren't always as clear as our intentions. There's an abundance of information out there. Not just on the internet but being spread from word to mouth. And with that much knowledge being passed around, there is bound to be some misinformation in the mix too. Not to mention, what's best for your coworker may not be best for you. What helps Mary Sue in Yoga Class lose weight in a week may not fit your schedule or desires. This might not be your first time reading about a weight loss method. Heck, you can be an absolute guru when it comes to the different diets out there. But where it all starts is at the basics of nutrition. What we will cover in this chapter is some key information that even your armchair nutritionist may not know. The hope is that next time someone whips out a comment on counting Calories, you'll be able to drop some fresh knowledge on them. Fresh as the veggies they seem to love.

Speaking of basics, it's important that we know what calories are exactly. "Calories" are a term used in the science of all forms, not just the healthy kind. It's used for measuring the amount of heat needed to consume a form of fuel. Sort of like how much heat is needed to burn coal to power an old-timey train engine. Though a lot cleaner in our case. When it comes to our bodies, we use it to measure the energy it takes for our metabolism to breakdown what we eat. If we are talking about Calories in food, we're really referring to how much energy your body is taking in. Little known fact, there's a bunch of different types of calories, like the "small calorie" or "gram calorie". This type of calorie is specifically referring to how much heat it takes to warm a gram of water. And in nutrition, what we call a "Calorie" is 1,000 small calories. That's why you will occasionally hear it referred to as a kilocalorie, but that's for the science types. Still, it's good to know that when you're reading a label and it says "10 Calories", it's shorthand for 10,000 small calories. Looks a lot more intimidating, doesn't it? Nutrition labels provide this term as a tool for all of us, so we know exactly how much energy you are gaining when eating different foods, and exactly how much we'll need to do to get rid of them efficiently. In short, your body consumes calories to keep your heart pumping and your brain sharp. Without them, you wouldn't survive.

But what we really want to know is how to burn Calories, and fast. One thing to keep in mind is that you need to burn more Calories than you are consuming. Sounds daunting aloud, but less so when put into context. Let's focus on the burn though. Exercise is one of the more obvious answers to getting rid of Calories. When you move, your body produces heat and that heat is a vital part of the process that is used to convert Calories into the required energy that sustains it. How you move determines how much energy is needed, and your body makes use of Calories to supply that energy. So, the more you move, the more Calories you use. It goes deeper than that though. Sometimes being active is just the best way to help your body be effective. When you move continuously for extended periods of time, your body requires more energy to sustain it, and down go the Calories. But different exercises can burn

Calories differently. Weight lifting, for example, will not burn nearly as many Calories as saying swimming or jogging. To expand on that fact, sprinting can burn more calories than jogging, but you can't do it for as long. Let's say someone weighs about 72 kilograms, that's about 160 pounds. If that person lifts free weights for one hour, they're going to burn 252 Calories. When that same person goes jogging for an hour, the results are doubled. They end up burning around 504 Calories. That's why it's commonly known that Cardio, or Cardiovascular exercise, is a top method to burn Calories and lose weight. But why is Cardio more efficient at burning Calories? Well, that has to do with metabolic rates and metabolism.

You see, when you perform cardiovascular exercises, you're raising your heart rate. You're getting that blood pumping. You're taking in tons of oxygen at higher speeds, and this lends a hand to your Metabolism. You've likely heard people talk about their Metabolism before, probably while complaining. They'll say things like it is too slow and that's why they can't lose weight. That is because Metabolism is the key process through which your body takes the foods you eat, converts them into Calories, and then turns those Calories into energy. And a key component of this is oxygen. So, while Cardio is making your heart pound, you are breathing harder and providing your Metabolism with more oxygen to help you utilize those Calories. That's why exercises like jogging are great for increasing your metabolic rate. And why exercises that don't require much breathing are not going to burn as many Calories. Earlier I mentioned how many Calories someone would burn in a certain situation. If you had an itch to know how much you'd shed while jogging, the way to find out is easy as a small equation!

You'll need your computer or phone handy for a bit of research, keep that in mind. First, determine your weight in kilograms. 2.2 pounds is about 1 kilogram, so someone that weighs 120 pounds is going to weigh 54.4 kilograms. An individual that weighs 200 pounds is going to measure at approximately 90.7 Kg. You can also just make use of the handy-dandy internet and plug the numbers into a search bar. Now you want to find the MET value of the exercise you are performing. Lists of these values can be found all over the internet, so it might take a quick google search. MET stands for

Metabolic Equivalent, which is a ratio of your metabolic rate while active to your metabolic rate while at rest. Again, more science, if you're into that. So, let's get an example! Say you ride your bike to work every day. Your commute is one hour, and your bike under 10 miles per hour. Taking it nice and easy. A leisurely bike ride like this is labeled by the MET as a 4.0, according to the 2011 Compendium. Now you just take your weight in Kg and multiply it by the 4.0 value. Say someone weighs the 54.4 kilograms mentioned earlier. The equation would be 54.4 x 4.0, which mean they worked off about 218 Calories if you round up. What's important to know about this equation is that it's based off a full hour of exercise. That means if you want to know how many Calories you shredded while sprinting for 30 minutes, you'll have to divide the results by 2. And if you want to know how much you burnt off from doing 15 minutes of laps in the pool, divide the results by 4.

Of course, everything can change depending on your metabolic rate. A lot of variables can be used to determine how your metabolism functions. Your sex, weight, height, and age are all deciding factors.

Woman, on average, need fewer Calories to maintain their body's functions. Older men have a slower metabolism than younger women. How many Calories you burn, how fast you burn them, and it's almost like the source code or the master key. Knowing how your metabolism operates is so vital to know how you should diet, exercise, or fast, that I strongly encourage you to take this time to calculate your metabolic rate. Figuring it out is just another equation, though this one might be easier if you just plug it into a computer. The proper name for BMR is Basal Metabolic Rate. If you're wondering, Basal stands for the base. It calculates the number of Calories needed to maintain your day-to-day body functions. You know, things like breathing and your heart pumping. There is also a term called RMR, or Resting Metabolic Rate, which is used interchangeably with the Basal Metabolic Rate, though slightly different in meaning. To calculate the BMR, you would use the Harris-Benedict Equation. The equation shifts numbers slightly, depending on if you are a man or a woman.

- For Women: 447.593 + (9.247 x Your Weight in Kg) + (3.098 x Your Height in centimeters) – (4.330 x Age)

- For Men: 88.362 + (13.397 x Your Weight in Kg) + (4.799 x Your Height in cm) – (5.677 x Age)

This can be someone what complex, so I'll include an example to get a feel of it. Let's just say someone weighs 68.039 kilograms. And yes, every number is important. They are a man and they stand at about 167.65 centimeters in height. This hypothetical man is 35 years old. The equation would look something like this.

- Harris-Benedict Equation for Men: 88.362 + (13.397 x 68.039 Kg) + (4.799 x 167.65 cm) – (5.677 x 35) = 1,605.7 Calories

It seems Mister Hypothetical here burns about 1,606 Calories just by living his life! Not too shabby. Now, you deserve to know that there is no way to calculate your metabolic rate down to a "T", as they say. These are just tools to help you estimate how many Calories you burn without performing any day-to-day activity like walking or exercising. It's certainly helpful to know this number, but even lab tests can't get it exactly right. Not to mention they are pretty darn expensive and time-consuming. But you can use this estimate of your Basal, or Base, Metabolic Rate to help keep you under that Calorie count. Or even combine it with the Calories you burn off through exercise. Say you BMR is 1,606 Calories, like Mister Hypothetical up there. And you ride your bike to work every day, a one-hour commute. Let's use that MET based equation from before. 68.039 Kg x 4.0 (MET) = 272.156 Calories burned. Wow! By riding his bike to work every day, Mister Hypothetical upped his metabolic rate to 1,878 Calories in a single day. And that's the value of these equations, both the MET Calorie Calculator and the Harris-Benedict Equation. You can use them anywhere as a guiding point. Whether it's for dieting, counting calories, exercising or fasting, I am positive these tools will make your health journey a smoother one.

We've talked about what Calories are, we've talked about how exercise helps get rid of them, but why diet then? Why not just exercise the Calories away, and eat whatever you'd like? Well, that has to do with the different foods you get Calories from. Your Metabolism is working hard to break down what you give it, but certain forms of food are more difficult to use as fuel than others. Starchy foods like kinds of pasta, rice, processed loaves of bread are especially complex and usually take the longest to be converted into fuel for your body. And that means they're going to sit inside of you for a longer time, turning into fats. We don't want that. We want our body breaking everything down and turning into energy as soon as possible. The less time it sits around, the less likely it will become pesky fat. Yes, there is a lot of talks out there about counting Calories and plenty of ways to get rid of them, but it isn't always about how many Calories you consume. Sometimes where you get those Calories from is far more important.

From Vegan to Keto, Paleo to the Mediterranean, there are so many ways you can eat. Let's be honest, it can be a bit daunting. And not every diet is right for everyone, so make sure to consider the nutrients your body needs most. Keto is one of the most popular diets around now. Health experts have raved about it, mainly because of how unique it is. Celebrities and athletes have used it, and it has a deep history. In these ways, it shares a lot with fasting. Keto is short for Ketogenic, and it's about reducing the carbohydrates and increasing fat intake. Sounds a bit contradictory to losing fat, but it works. The goal is to send your body into a state Ketosis, getting it accustomed to using fats as fuel. Which means that your body will start targeting the fat deposits and breaking them down. It's also quite difficult because you need to avoid all sugars and carbs, including the hidden ones. All diets have their own challenges though. With Keto, you eat healthy fats because they're the easiest for your body to breakdown into fuel. Foods like avocados and coconuts, oily fish, and some nuts are in this diet. But why is this so important? Because, instead of having to break down carbohydrates, turn them into sugars, and then turn those sugars into fuel, you're cutting out the middle man. Simple, unrefined foods are always the easiest to breakdown. Especially ones high in fats and low in sugars. It's a common thread to eating healthy.

Another popular diet you may have heard of is the Mediterranean diet, which highlights the nutritional habits of people living in the Mediterranean region. These are the folk from Southern Europe. We're talking Greece, Southern Italy, and even Crete. Spain and

France also fall in that category. And again, this diet focuses on cutting out a lot of refined foods and carbohydrates, replacing them with easily converted alternatives. Eggs, grains, and seeds, cheeses, fish and poultry. The common themes between all diets are that you are replacing what is not easily processed with more natural substitutes. And of course, the golden rule. Avoid carbs, avoid sugars, as your life depends on it! It's a common misconception that going on a diet means cutting out your favorite snacks and treats, but it really means shifting where you get your nutrients from. You can still eat desserts, just ones that your body can make use of. That way, your metabolism can become more efficient, converting food into Calories in the blink of an eye.

If different foods can help your metabolism, how does not eating foods help? What does fasting do? It might seem obvious that consuming fewer Calories than you are burning will help you lose weight. We all know that. But the helpful effects of fasting can go far beyond this. Like eating different types of food, eating foods at different times can help your body in several ways. The body's metabolism can move faster and make the most out of the nutrients you're feeding it. In many ways, you can lose weight fast, no pun intended. With great results and less dodging food groups, it can be the way to go for many individuals who are looking to kick a certain amount of weight in a specific amount of time. In fact, intermittent fasting is very popular with celebrities and models for that very reason. They love using it to slim down as quick as can be, and most have established it as their preferred method of weight management, even after cutting weight for the next role. You'll hear super healthy people like Terry Crews and Hugh Jackman, talk all about it. Do you remember Wolverine? Well, he uses the intermittent fast.

Is intermittent fasting different from your average diet though? Will you lose more weight, will it help you build muscle tone? Is it that much better than eating certain foods? There are so many questions bouncing around. And the majority of answers to those questions are "Yes." And the reason is this; you can lose as much weight with just intermittent fasting as you can from dieting and working out. This means you're doing less to get the same results. On top of that, you can eat your regular food groups, so long as you're not eating them when you're supposed to be fasting. The real trick is being consistent. Of course, avoiding those carbs and super sugary foods helps as well. Unlike diets like Keto, where you must follow a strict diet that allows zero room for error, you have all the freedom in the world to eat as you like and still find yourself achieving the same goal. To lose weight. There is no fancy state you're tricking your body into, though there is a bunch of sound science to back it all up. I know, it's hard to believe. You're probably asking yourself if it's too good to be true. "All I have to do is skip my morning meal? How is this possible? And why have celebrities been keeping their secrets from us?" Well, I don't have all the answers, but I can tell you not eating breakfast is harder than it sounds. We do have some great tips later that can help you get into the habit though, so just hang on.

Let's look at what it will be like to lose 1 kilogram. Not a lot, I know, but it's a start! The experts tell us that a single pound of fat is roughly 3,500 Calories to burn. We know that you lose weight by consuming fewer calories than you are burning through the day. This is called creating a caloric deficit. Don't be intimidated by the big words, it is much easier than it sounds. So, we want to lose about one pound. Let's give ourselves about a week to do it. That's not too hard, so long as you're smart about how you eat, or when. If you create a deficit of about 500 to 700 Calories a day, you'll be well on your way to losing that pound. If you stick to the higher side of that number, you'll be closer to burning a pound and a half off. But what about a single kilogram? That takes a bit more work, so let's set the goal for one kilogram burned in two weeks. Since one kilogram is 2.2 pounds, you'll want to double those numbers. And if you keep to the goal you set, you'll have no trouble kicking that kilo. Over that two-week span, you need a caloric deficit of about 7,700 Calories! Sounds like a big number, but not if you break it down over the fourteen days. That's only 550 Calories a day, easily achieved by a walk around the block after dinner. Let's call on Mister Hypothetical for our example here. Based on the Harris-Benedict Equation, we know that he burns 1,606 Calories in a day, without any activity included. If he eats four eggs with cheese for breakfast, that's 561 Calories. Mister Hypothetical is dieting though, so he'll be exchanging that sandwich for a nice grilled chicken salad with bacon and ranch. That's another 247 Calories. He'll only drink water through the day that keeps his Calorie count low. And he's feeling adventurous tonight. He's had a long day, walking around the office collecting spreadsheets. So now he wants some to jazz up his dinner. Mister Hypothetical throws a chicken breast into the skillet, with some mushrooms and spinach to give it some great flavor. That's another 257 Calories! And wouldn't you know it, his caloric deficit for the day is 541 Calories. He does that for seven days in a row and now he's reached his goal of burning one pound a week, and then some. Does it two weeks in a row? Now Mister Hypothetical has let go of a whole kilogram of fat. Congratulations, Hypothetical. You're off to a great start.

What if Mister Hypothetical preferred fasting over dieting? One type of intermittent fasting is 16/8 fast. There a bunch of different forms of fasting, but this one is most common and is spoken highly of. If you want to know other kinds of fast, don't worry. We'll be going into detail about this. For now, Mister Hypothetical decides to eat from noon to 5 pm. This is the 8 in the 16/8 fast. He skips his breakfast and has a light snack of grapes, about 100 grams of them, a little over a cup when noon rolls around. At lunch, around 3 pm, he has an egg sandwich with mayo, and that holds him over for a little while longer. No skipping the sandwich today, Mister Hypothetical. You're starting to see how fasting comes into play. By just glossing over breakfast, which is usually heavy in Calories, and having his snack at work, he's saved himself a bunch of room on his caloric deficit. 67 Calories for grapes, 390 Calories for the egg sandwich, and only two hours left to eat a final meal. Mister Hypothetical isn't starving though, he just ate a couple of hours ago. So, what does he do? He grabs a milkshake, which tosses on 350 Calories, and calls it a day. That's awesome, right? Getting to have a dessert at the end of the night? So how does Mister Hypothetical measure up in his caloric deficit while fasting? Our fellow health enthusiast is at a whopping 799! Compared to the 541 caloric deficit he achieved while eating healthy? He's burning 2,093 Calories more a week that while he was dieting. And he got to have some dessert. Keep in mind that these numbers are based off the Basal Metabolic Rate, so if he's walking around the office, strolling down the road to get lunch, or even running to catch a train, he's burning 60 to 100 Calories more a day. At the end of the 14 days, Mister

Hypothetical cut out 11,000 Calories while fasting, losing closer to two kilograms than just one. Meanwhile, dieting only helped him cut 7,500 Calories if he kept at his pace of four eggs a day at breakfast. And he didn't even get to have dessert. Now we're really starting to see the benefits of fasting compared to dieting.

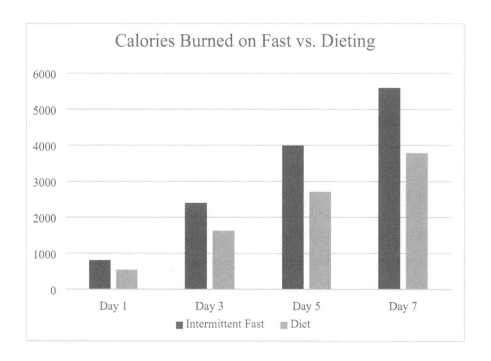

So now you know all you possibly can about why people diet. How Calories work, what burning them off really takes, isn't rocket science. Yet, with so many options out there, I'm sure it will help for you to have this quick guide in your back pocket. Want to know how your exercises helped in cutting those Calories down? Pull out the MET key and punch in those numbers. Curious on what you're burning while you sit there and read this book? Pull up the Harris-Benedict Equation and you'll have your answers. You know there are different diets that may work for you, and some that might not. Different foods you can eat to help boost your metabolism. And not just that, you know why they can boost your metabolic rate. That's a lot more important and even more helpful. Next time someone in the office brings up their diet, you can discuss with them if they are taking in too many foods with complex sugars, and maybe even suggest a healthier alternative. But what's really covered here, is why you picked up this book. The answers you've been looking for. Confirming all your doubts about dieting, and all your hopes about fasting. We see clear benefits of intermittent fasting when compared to your average diet. Taking all of this in, it's evident why so many celebrities, models, and doctors recommend intermittent fasting as a healthy alternative to strict dieting, while still maintaining a normal lifestyle. It permits you to burn the Calories and lose weight while enjoying a milkshake at the end of your night. And we've only begun to scratch the surface!

Chapter 2: The Importance of Fasting

Where did fasting come from? It's not as if it appeared out of the blue. Like I mentioned earlier, fasting has its roots deeply embedded in our history. From spiritual practices to health practices, we see that it has been discussed and studied for thousands of years. It's incredibly important to development as a civilization. And while so many people believe that the earliest records of it were strictly boasted as a spiritual practice that is a myth. In fact, fasting, in general, has always been considered a method for cleansing the body of toxins and healing it. Of course, the debate has taken place over whether spiritual and physical healing has often been conflated or confused. Yet, with so much popularity and attention thrown onto this healthy method of weight loss, sound science is coming out that backs up the claims of icons from our past. I will be covering some of this research and the results below. But first, I'd like to highlight how integral fasting has been in shaping our world. In fact, we are hard pressed to find a single recorded time in human history where people did not fast.

Within Ancient societies, fasting was especially revered for its abundant health benefits. Among them were "cleansing impurities from the body" and "bringing an acute clarity to the mind." Countless names through our history have proclaimed fasting as their biggest tools. Some of those names belong to people we revere to this day. The renowned Greek mathematician Pythagoras was an early advocate of fasting. If you've picked up a math book, you know of him. But what they didn't teach you in math class, is how crucial fasting was in his studies. Not only did he believe it had numerous health benefits, he vouched that it also augmented the mind's creativity. One could theorize that some of the greatest discoveries of the past were facilitated through fasting. In fact, this genius of the old world fasted for a full 40 days! But don't worry, we're not going to recommend taking it that far. So passionately did he advocate for this practice, that he also made each of his students fast before attending his teachings. And he wasn't the only wise man, or woman, of the past who spoke of fasting. It's incredibly popular with Greek intellectuals. Plato spoke of medical practices that were considered "false" and "true", separating them. And in the category of truth fell fasting. It was Hippocrates, the Father of Modern Medicine himself, who spoke of fasting no longer being a simple philosophical practice. The healing process of fasting was referred to as the "Inner Physician."

"Everyone has a physician inside him or her; we just have to help it in its work. The natural healing force within each one of us is the greatest force in getting well. Our food should be our medicine. Our medicine should be our food. But to eat when you are sick is to feed your sickness." – Hippocrates

---

We also see great minds like Plutarch, the Biographer and Essayist, speak on fasting. "Instead of using a medicine, rather, fast a day." Of course, we're not recommending that you stop taking your prescription. Yet there is strong evidence to support the claims of these teachers. However, the point is that some of the brightest minds in this world knew how helpful fasting was for good health, both physically and mentally. And this was centuries ago! Other well-known figures who we know fasted are:

- Confucius
- Leonardo da Vinci
- Socrates
- Lao-Tzu
- Seneca

And the list goes on. It is evident that across the entire world, and throughout history, the keenest of intellectuals supported fasting. We're talking about individuals who have shaped the world as we know it. But the importance of fasting has gone far beyond physical and spiritual cleansing. Only a handful of years ago, it became a popular method of peaceful protest. The Suffragettes, who have helped our world find a balance and sense of equality, led hunger strikes in the early 20th Century. July 1909, Marion Wallace-Dunlop fasted for her rights and the rights of her sisters. She was arrested multiple times for speaking out against the oppression of women. Cesar Chavez, Mexican American union leader, fasted for fair wages and treatment for farm workers. And perhaps the most famous among these activists, Mahatma Gandhi, fasted in absolute protest of Britain's colonial rule of India. It's evident that fasting hasn't just shaped our world's spiritual beliefs. Fasting has influenced medicine, philosophy, science, and politics.

Monks do it, political leaders do it, heck, and you may have even done it. Probably without realizing it. The point here is that fasting is not some mysterious subject. It is a practice that has been observed a thousand times over by the leaders of our world. You may find individuals that say we don't know the results of fasting. This is simply not true. There are numerous studies on the subject, ancient and current. Some skeptics say that this method may not provide your body with the proper nutrients it needs to run in tip-top shape. This is also not true. If it were, I am sure that celebrities and models, people our society considers the height of physical appeal, would not be going along with it. It's been a technique of fitness trainers for years, and a lot of stars love speaking out about how it's revolutionized their weight loss methods. Mainly because you can cut so many Calories, without touching the weights. Since it is a practice that has been observed throughout history, in many different peoples around the globe, we know it works. We're confident in that fact. And there is an abundance of scientific standing behind what they spoke of in the past. Here's a name we all may know. Chris Pratt is very outspoken about fasting for his health. Daniel, a prophet from the Bible, fasted to get closer to God. Chris Pratt uses the "Daniel Fast" to lose weight and deepen his connection with his body. 21 days without meat, animal products, bread, and processed foods. Of course, this is a very intense method of fasting, but not the only kind. Another star admired for his health would be Chris Hemsworth, better known as Thor, or the God of Thunder. This guy uses the intermittent fast anytime he's trying to lose wait for a role, and he's been doing it as far back as 2013. And the list of celebrities that use the intermittent fast goes on.

- Beyoncé
- Justin Theroux
- Nicole Kidman
- Antoni Porowski
- Jennifer Lopez
- Miranda Kerr
- Benedict Cumberbatch
- Ben Affleck

This list can fill an entire page, but I don't want to waste your time reading off names. It is worth noting that there are also some athletes who use intermittent fasting to give them an edge. Georges St-Pierre, for one! A Canadian Mixed Martial Artist, who is considered one of the greatest fighters in MMA history. This man has a single meal a day, and he isn't the only one. You may have heard of Wim Hof as an extreme athlete of Dutch origin that has set multiple Guinness World Records. He's achieved remarkable feats like "Swimming Under Ice" and "Prolonged Full-body Contract with Ice". And Hof still holds the record for running a barefoot half-marathon on ice and snow. He also only eats one meal a day! Can you imagine doing all that while only eating lunch? So, whether fasting works to calm the inner turmoil of your soul, or calm your worries about fitting into that swimsuit, is just a matter of perspective. It can push you to amazing feats like these athletes or help you establish a discipline most people crave in their lives. The only real mystery here is how fasting helps your body in so many ways.

But why do these individuals use fasting over dieting? Well, for one, it can be far faster. Namely, because you're eating a fraction of the Calories you'd consume, even when diets. Chose the One Meal a Day fast, like the athletes mentioned earlier. You could have a full course meal, and still, barely touch the Calorie count of a three-course diet meal. Say you're going to have four chicken thighs baked in the oven, a side of broccoli with butter, and a slice of apple pie for dessert. Alright, the golden rule says no carbs, but what if this is your cheat day? The four thighs are about 360 Calories, the broccoli with butter is 140, and the dessert is 296. That means your one meal a day plan has you at 796 Calories. But what if you wanted three healthy diet meals, no carbs? Say you have turkey sausage, peppers, and onions for breakfast. Sounds pretty good, right? Well, that's 350 Calories, first thing in the morning. You have a Caesar Salad with Chicken & Bacon for lunch, and that's another 320 Calories. And at dinner time? You get home and cook yourself a chicken breast with brussels sprouts, which tacks on another 510 Calories. Add that all together, and even with your three meals a day you're consuming a total of 1,180 Calories. So, you can see why weight loss coaches and celebrities prefer to only eat for a portion of the day. Even with a dessert, your caloric deficit is vastly superior when you do an intermittent fast. This gives you a lot more wiggle room while helping you blow your goals right out of the water. 800 Calories a day, which is very doable through the intermittent fasting method, and you're burning at least 5,000 Calories in a week. 1,200 Calories a day, you're burning a little over half of what you might be fasting. About 2,800 Calories in a week. That's close to two pounds burned in a week, compared to under one pound dropped through dieting. As you can see, fasting done right blows weight loss diets out of the water. And with none of the fancy dodging, you have to do with diets like Keto. This, coupled with the fact that fasting helps your metabolism burn more Calories a day, makes it obvious why there's a list of over 40 stars out there who prefer fasting to dieting.

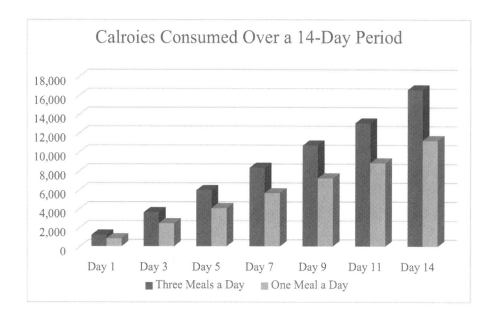

Calroies Consumed Over a 14-Day Period

Now we've covered how fasting is important to our history as a people. We've talked about how and why it is constantly used by icons relevant to this century, rather than dieting. But how is it important for our health? Fasting will certainly help you lose a ton of weight, no doubt about that. So, for just a few moments, I'd like to touch on some of the more fascinating discoveries intermittent fasting research has revealed in the last century. As I mentioned, the power of fasting only begins with weight loss. And before I go through how exactly it does this, let's cover some of the additional benefits you'll receive through fasting. In fact, you deserve to know exactly what the unintended by-products of this lifestyle will be. And don't worry, they're all very exciting. I firmly believe that, by knowing these effects ahead of time, you'll be far more enthused to start your fast. You'll probably gain an unexpected conviction, a dedication even, to this new life. You'll certainly understand why men and women remembered thousands of years down the line of history all advocated for this health practice of intermittent fasting.

There are modern medical studies on intermittent fasting dating back to 1945. The study I am referencing was done with mice in a lab and yielded surprising results. Though they wouldn't be so surprising to the likes of ancient physicians. "The optimum amount of fasting appeared to be fasting one day in three, and this increased the life span of littermate males about 20% and littermate females about 15%." This was recorded in *The Journal of Nutrition*, Volume 31, and Issue 3, published on the 1st of March 1946. It was released under the names of Anton J. Carlson and Frederick Hoelzel. Carlson was a Swedish American physiologist, well known for his works, such as *The Control of Hunger in Health and Disease* (University of Chicago Press, 1916). Another study released more recently, January

9th, 2006, mentions even more impressive results. It states that, through restricting caloric intake by means of alternate day fasts, research has revealed to us that fasting "...extends lifespan 30-50% and confers near perfect health across a broad range of species." The experiments had been performed since May 2003, over the course of a three-year testing period. This report is titled "The Effect on Health of Alternate Day Calorie Restriction: Eating Less and More than Needed on Alternate Days Prolongs Life", and was released by James B. Johnson, Donald R. Laub, and Sujit John. It is published in *Medical Hypotheses*, Volume 67, and Issue 2. And by looking at this study, it's no surprise that Pythagoras was believed to have been 75 to 100 years old at the time of his death. Meanwhile, the average Greek only lived to be about 35-40 years of age!

The discoveries found in these reports do not stop there, elaborating on the fact that fasting is a crucial tool in preventing and managing various diseases.

This process was likely formed by evolution. In "The Effect on Health of Alternate Day Calorie Restriction" they speak about some of the things found to be resisted and treated through Intermittent Fasting.

Medical conditions such as asthma and seasonal allergies. They mark resistance to infectious diseases of viral, bacterial and fungal origin (URIs, recurrent bacterial tonsillitis, chronic sinusitis, periodontal disease). Autoimmune disorders, such as rheumatoid arthritis and osteoarthritis was additionally found to be relieved in test subjects. Furthermore, they mention the symptoms of CNS inflammatory lesions, like Tourette's syndrome and Meniere's disease, are a lesson as well. Different forms of Cardiac Arrhythmias, or irregular heartbeats, like PVCs and atrial fibrillation, are found to be likewise soothed through fasting. The doctors who authored this research even bring up a resistance to hot flashes caused by menopause. The professionals then make a hypothesis, stating that there is a belief among them that many other conditions could be improved, delayed, and possibly even prevented. Conditions like congestive heart failure, brain injury due to thrombotic stroke atherosclerosis, multiple sclerosis, and NIDDM. Even Alzheimer's and Parkinson's are theorized to be prevented or relieved through an intermittent fasting treatment.

I know, a lot of complex words and detailed findings. The point these professionals are trying to make is that a wide array of conditions and health complications found in our modern age can be treated or prevented. Through calorie restrictions like intermittent fasting, a large portion of the issues we face as Americans eating three meals a day can be avoided entirely. That is why it comes as no surprise that many of these diseases and conditions are caused by an excess of consumption, which can and will result in a buildup of toxins in our bodies. Yet, a quick google search says that detoxification of the body through fasting is a myth. If this is the case, why do we find several reports and research papers from around the world, typically outside of America, that says differently? Studies from medical professionals, detailing the successful treatment of illness and disease that is believed to come from excess toxins in the bloodstream. Or in the case of one research study, a compromised immune system resulting in the inflammatory skin condition known as atopic dermatitis. This study was performed in Kyung Hee Medical Center of Korea and supervised by Doctor Kyu Seok Kim as well as Doctor Hae Jeong Nam, from March 2010 to February of 2012. The findings are published in the article "Detoxification Combining Fasting with Fluid Therapy for Refractory Cases of Severe Atopic Dermatitis". I would like to first highlight a statement within this report. "Westernized medicine has conventionally used a combination of practices that make it difficult for long-term treatment and may endanger the life of the subject." This gives us an idea of why Western medicine refutes any possibility of fasting being able to treat and detoxify the body. They have practices that are costly and believed to be effective. However, in the article, they discuss how difficult continuous use of this treatment is on patients, namely due to side effects. And so fasting combined with fluid therapy is investigated as an alternative. The results were quite telling. They discuss how fasting for certain periods of time can diminish irritation with the gastrointestinal tract, eliminate body waste, and while refreshing digestive and respiratory organs. This can be especially helpful for patients whose AD is seemingly aggravated by allergens, or toxins, within foods as they are being digested. The fasting and fluid therapy helped relieve them of symptoms. It is believed that where the body's normal detoxifying functions fail, the fasting and fluid therapy augmented the process and provided the extra detoxification necessary to drive out impurities. "A low-energy diet reduced inflammatory symptoms and oxidative damage in patients with AD."

Simply put, western medicine does not consider toxins as a result of excessive food intake. They talk about toxins as something that invades your body, mainly through the air you breathe. However, numerous cases are coming out in medicine countering this. Studies that are confirming that many diseases arise from a buildup of waste from excess food consumption. That waste becomes toxins that can influence your health negatively. Especially when combined with the synthetic chemicals and preservatives in so much of what we eat and drink. Certainly, your body can detoxify naturally. When you are not over-consuming. Doctor Alan Goldhamer also mentions the conflict of Western Medicine with results seen in fasting practices. In the following quote, Doctor Goldhamer is talking about what he witnessed while attending Pacific College in Australia.

"There, I had a chance to see what

*happens when you do anything
intelligently or use fasting appropriately.
And it was pretty mind-bending. So, I
saw a lot of people who I had to been
trained to not get well, get well, and they
did that consistently through the use of
fasting..." – Doctor Alan Goldhamer,
Founder and Education Director of
TrueNorth Health Center*

In *Ageing Research Reviews*, Volume 39, released in October of 2017, researches elaborated on this discussion. The report is titled "Impact of Intermittent Fasting on Health and Disease Processes". In the last century of our world, overconsumption and excess have become a notable problem, especially in first world countries. In the past, animals and humans did not have access to such an abundance of food and resources. This may be why, perhaps by some grand design, we have evolved to function in a far more efficient manner when we are deprived of food or left in a fasting state. In physiological research and studies, fasting refers to a metabolic state when a person has not eaten for an extended period. This state usually appears when you don't eat overnight and can also be reached once 8-12 hours have gone by since your last meal. The first changes in metabolism can be noted within 3-5 hours after eating. Science has observed that these changes can take place both in your physical body and your cognitive processes. Just like the Greek teachers said, you can become more creative and more perceptive when you fast. The authors of the research above, go on to say something relatively remarkable. Intermittent fasting triggers an adaptive cellular stress response. This is the primary factor that contributes to cellular and molecular methods of counteracting disease and improving health. The signal pathways in your brain and this has given birth to amazing phenomena. Events such as a marked enhancement in mitochondrial health, the DNA in our bodies literally being repaired, strand by strand. We discover the process of Autophagy being augmented. If you are wondering what Autophagy has to do with anything, it is a function that takes place within every cell in our bodies. Our cells have developed a very natural, and regulated system over years of evolution. When a cell discovers components within and labels them as unnecessary or dysfunctional, Autophagy begins. These components are either recycled or degrade in a very organic manner. It's a miraculous system and is part of what the ancient teachers were observing when they noticed fasting helping people who are diseased or sick. When scientific studies are discovering the effects of fasting on various diseases, Autophagy has a huge role to play in all of this. The cells are sent into a sensitive state, which can speed up the process of autophagy. Isn't it the body fascinating? The fact that what has been theorized and discussed throughout history is now defined through scientific knowledge. Your body really does have an "inner physician", as Hippocrates discussed. It's always been there, and it is called autophagy. That is why intermittent fasting and partial fasting can help suppress the symptoms of many diseases and can even prevent the contraction of them.

Going back to the research we were discussing earlier, there is another fascinating event that takes place in subjects who take advantage of intermittent and partial fasting. Stem cell-based regeneration. Stem cells have gained a heightened level of attention within the last few decades. But what are they exactly? In biology, stem cells are labeled as an undefined cell within organisms with multicellular composition. We, humans, fall under this category, which you learned back in your high school biology class. These cells can support and create an infinite number of cells of the same origin. Not only that, they have the amazing ability to allow other cells of different types to arise from this replication, through several methods and processes that are being currently being discovered and researched. Stem cell science has come leaps and bounds, thanks to the heightened awareness and support communities are showing. Stem cells have already been used to treat diseases, right? Absolutely! Stem cells have been grown in labs and can also be transferred by donors. One method that transfers stem cells is a bone marrow transplant. Through a bone marrow transplant, stem cells can replace damaged cells, like those affected by chemotherapy. They can also be used to give the immune system a kick! This helps fight numerous forms of cancer and blood-related diseases. Lymphoma, leukemia, multiple myeloma, and even neuroblastoma. Most of these donor stem cells come from adults, though there is also the ability to use the umbilical cord blood for this.

I don't want to get too controversial, so I'll circle back to stem cell regeneration being discovered in those of us who are fasting. While it is not a known fact, many physicians and experts theorize that fasting can be used to treat and even defeat cancers, when combined with other medical practices. The research is still being carried out however, so we don't recommend you put all your eggs in one basket. However, it is not a far-fetched concept that, if your stem cell regeneration is rapidly increased by intermittent and partial fasting, it can be used to treat the body's most crippling enemies. Horrendous occurrences, like cancer and cellular degradation. And even if this is not 100% proven, the prevention of other diseases through IF (intermittent fasting) is. So, it doesn't hurt to give it a shot. But who knows? Just like the numerous health benefits of fasting were once believed to be pseudoscience and quackery, research may reveal that these theories are correct. One day, a sick individual may not need to get a stem cell transfer or take part in these controversial procedures. The pain and suffering of chemotherapy could even be a thing in the past. Better yet, they may not need to pay a dime to recover and beat the world's most deadly illnesses! The hope is that one day, you will simply be able to skip a meal or two, and your body does what is always meant to.

When it comes to this natural occurrence of stem cell regeneration and autophagy, research has shown that it can begin within mammals as soon as 24 to 48 hours of intermittent and partial fasting. And even sooner, if one fast for a whole day, or two days in a row. And what about the neurological effects of fasting? Well, in western medicine, we often only focus on symptoms. Not preventative measures. Though fasting is often discredited by popular American medicine, despite sound research supporting its numerous benefits that is not the case across seas. In fact, German researchers and scientists have always stood by fasting, while American and Western standards of medicine labeled it as nonsensical. In 2014, a German research article was released called "Metabolic and Psychological Response to 7-Day Fasting". This article provides an excellent insight into the effects of fasting on someone's psychological state. Those tested were allowed approximately 300 to 400 Calories a day. The researchers found that, over the two weeks of testing, there were notable psychological and mental results. "Fasting-induced mood enhancement was shown through decreased depression, fatigue, anxiety, and improved vigor." Let's focus deeper on some of the effects fasting had on balances in the brain. The people fasting were found to have a modified sleep architecture, which was likely a key contributor to the decrease in fatigue and the improvement of energy levels. This could also be tied to the increased metabolic rate, which allows for better use of the 300-400 Calories the subjects were consuming. The study also revealed that, by fasting, we're able to receive more frequent endorphin releases and an increased level of serotonin available to us.

"In evolutionary terms, enhancement of mood after a number of days experiencing food deprivation appears to be a vital psychological adaptation in the search for sustenance and the likelihood of survival."

And this increase in happiness is not restricted to just the seven days fast. Similar results have been found in prolonging testing through the Intermittent Fasting and Partial Fasting. As was stated earlier, the by-product of this new lifestyle choice is going to go well beyond your weight. You're not just going to lose weight easier;

you're going to feel better while doing it. You'll find yourself with more energy than you had before, which may surprise you. And with time, your body will resist the diseases and health problems you may have had before. The illnesses that your friends and family may be suffering from, you'll naturally be avoiding! And as you go on through life, you'll find yourself aging slower, thanks to the natural autophagy and stem cell regeneration that will take place through intermittent and partial fasting. As you can see, it is no wonder the teachers of our past lived so long. Their beliefs on fasting healing the body and cleansing the mind were sound. And the hope contained within this book is that you shall also experience a beautiful, vigorous life that is extended through this health practice. That your mind will be clear, your heart light, and your health impeccable. Now let's talk about what intermittent fasting is all about. Weight loss.

Chapter 3: What is Intermittent Fasting?

We've talked abundantly about fasting through history. Why it has been so important and been talked about so thoroughly, through history. Not just the obvious reasons, like doubling your weight loss goals compared to dieting. The secret ones too. The reasons that have made it a point of consideration of every advanced civilization known to this day. You're covered on all the obscure, unexpected boons to your health when it comes to fasting. Autophagy, stem cell regeneration, an extension on your life span, and a slower aging process. You can have a grand old time going back in for with some who says Veganism is better for than Fasting. List off some of those discoveries we covered, I guarantee their eyes will go wide. If they doubt you, make sure they know that there proven medical studies that back all of it up, released online. So now it's time to talk about why you're really reading this book. Intermittent fasting. The same health practice that helps create all those benefits we talked about above. The real meat and potatoes. By now, you're probably thrilled to know that by just skipping a few meals a week, you'll have such a dramatic increase in results. Almost double the amount of weight loss recorded through traditional diets. You're probably wondering how such a potent health practice have been passed down through the centuries, yet you're only now getting all the information. What is this Intermittent Fasting really?

Intermittent fasting is the broad name for weight loss methods where you fast to some degree. It can be fasting for a portion of the day, fasting every other day, or even fasting for a set number of days in the week, and eat on other days. There is a lot of diversity to this health practice. Yet intermittent fasting is seen to be vastly superior when compared to traditional fasting methods. We should avoid considering it or comparing it to a diet. A diet, by definition, is committing yourself to a specific set of food groups, and not breaking from that guide you set for yourself, using it as a means of weight loss. However intermittent fasting, as we discussed in the previous chapter, is not strictly used for weight loss. It's a helpful practice that has been used by peoples all throughout history and across the world to achieve a sound state of health. It does not restrict what foods you can eat and can even be used in compound with a specific diet. As far as weight loss goes, intermittent fasting is designed as a pattern of eating to get the most out of your meals. Remember the golden rule though, avoid carbs at all costs. That's a must to lose weight, no matter what method you are using.

So how is intermittent fasting different from your classic fast? Well, to explain that, we need to discuss the different types of traditional casting methods. There's a veritable plethora of them out there. And while they may help you for certain reasons, the results are significantly different than intermittent fasting. Let's start with the juice fast. It's very common, and unique. A juice fast is basically consuming exclusively liquids from different types of plants, vegetables, and fruits. No solid foods are eaten at any point. The average juice fast will last anywhere from one to two weeks, though some people take it above and beyond. While it's very straightforward, someone on a juice fast will want to plan for the period they'll be following this method. Why? Because you'll have to make sure you're getting more than enough vitamins and minerals while on the fast. Nutrients are essential to any weight loss method, which means you can't just drink onion and banana juice alone. So, what starts off sounding like a really simple weight loss method ends up being a lot more complex. You're trying to get that precise blend of fruits or veggies that give you all you need. Not to mention, fruits are notorious for their high sugar content. And since there is no real "limit" to how often you can consume these juices, it is very easy to slide down a path of drinking several sugary smoothies day after day. And four to six "juice meals" a day, each ranking at 400 to 500 Calories, can blow your caloric deficit out of the water. You'll be hard-pressed to burn off 2,000 – 2,400 Calories a day, especially when they're layered with sugars. It's important to note that this is just a fast in name since most of the time your body isn't going into the "fasting" state that yields the health benefits of intermittent and partial fasting.

Another popular fasting method is water fast. Very straightforward, and not too effective. Essentially, you'll be eliminating everything from your diet for 24 to 72 hours, though the really daring have been known to push it as far as a week. This isn't a liquid only fast, which we will cover soon. The water fast is strict to its name. Those who embark on this journey will be drinking at least two liters of water per day, though it is encouraged to try three liters instead. This makes up for the hydration you'd normally get from foods. Some of the benefits of water fast are rapid weight loss. Unfortunately, most of the weight you'll be losing is carbs that have been stored in your body and water weight. And while you may lose a noted amount of weight in a day, it'll come back as soon as you start eating again. This is due to your body's delay in burning the fat. Stored fats require at least three to four days before being consumed. This is the primary reason you'll hear the extremists talk about water fasting for a whole week. "The best way to get the most out of a water fast. None of the fake results." This is one of the many reasons intermittent fasting is recommended over these types of fasts. Yet water fasts do share a few of the benefits of healthy, prolonged fasting like the intermittent fast. Remember, it's never terrible for you to skip a day of eating and just drink lots of water. It helps flush your system. Though you're still better off with a researched and verified method, like IF (intermittent fasting).

Here is one of the more extreme fasting methods around, though it doesn't pose itself as one. The Master Cleanse. The diet was first created in the 1940s and gained a lot of popularity in the 70s when Stanley Burroughs published the book "The Master Cleanser". Stanley is the creator of this cleansing method, reported helping people shed weight fast. The basics of this diet are drinking six to 12 glasses of a "special lemonade" in a single day, plus a gallon of saltwater. The lemonade is a blend of lemon juice, maple syrup, water, and a pinch of cayenne pepper. And they take it one step further by recommending you drink an herbal laxative tea as part of this weight loss method. Supposedly this drink will be enough to give you your nutrients through the day, thanks to the "rich source of vitamins and minerals" in lemons and maple syrup? People who subscribe to this method must begin their day with a salt water flush. As time goes on, they drink their several cups of lemonade and end it all with their cup of laxative tea. Apparently, you do this anywhere from 10 to 40 days, and you'll lose insane amounts of weight. Anyone who is this desperate to lose weight should really consider safer methods because the Master Cleanse is proven to be unhealthy. Not only do you get nowhere near enough nutrients for your body, but you're also consuming an excessive amount of sugar and the weight loss you achieved never remains. In fact, it can come back remarkably quick, thanks to the effects the "Master Cleanse" has on your metabolism. A. k. a. throwing it all out of whack. Beyoncé once used this method. Now she uses intermittent fasting. Is there any wonder why?

Let's discuss another type of fast, which is none too different from the others. It's known as the liquid fast. And like the juice fast, you can consume all your nutrients in liquid form. The only real difference is you allowed to drink liquids other than juice. Coffee, tea, milkshakes, it doesn't matter. If it's liquid, it counts. And like the juice fast, it's a misnomer. There is no real fasting involved because the body never gets a break. A lot of people do crazy things with this "fast", including cooking different foods then blending them? And while it can certainly yield some health benefits, those who choose this practice will rarely lose any weight at all. And like these other fasts, once you go back to eating, most of the weight comes back. So long as you're willing to drink eggs and veggie smoothies for the rest of your life, there's no problem.

And last, but not least, is the Daniel Fast. Remember Chris Pratt and his fast from the last chapter? Well, this is it. One of the more hardcore methods of fasting, that last 21 days. Essentially, for the 21 days, you are using this fast, you can only eat certain groups of food. These include foods with plant oils, whole grain, seeds, nuts, legumes, vegetables, and fruits. It's essentially caloric restriction like partial fasting and intermittent fasting. Out of all the facts listed above, this one has revealed health benefits closest to those observed in the research of intermittent fasting that was covered earlier. Most notably, an improvement of the factors tied to cardiovascular and metabolic disease. If you're feeling like trying multiple methods of fasting, and you're experienced with long term fasting already, this method wouldn't be too harsh for you. The biggest thing to remember is that it takes more commitment than your typical intermittent fast.

Looking at the results of these practices, it is no surprise a lot of people think all fasting falls under the "fad diet" category. Some of these are just plain diets, and most aren't even really fasting. They're posing under the last name, so as to throw people off the fact that you are just dieting. Almost all of them are seen to be misguided attempts of losing weight in a very short period through excessive methods. With concepts like the juice fast and the "Master Cleanse" being thrown into the category of IF, you can see why people bash it. That's why it is necessary for you to know what fasting really is, and what it is not. These wild practices are often extremely unhelpful in weight loss, confuse your body, and can really be detrimental to your health. The safest of these methods would be water fasting and the Daniel Fast, which some would argue falls under the label of a partial fast, though with more restrictions.

What is the difference between intermittent fasting compared to these methods? Well, for one, it's not pseudo-fasting. Intermittent and partial fasting is the real deal. And if we want to have a firm grasp on what a true fast is, and how it aids in fat loss, we first need to wrap our mind around the state this method puts your body in. You see, when you consume food, especially three times a day, your body is constantly left in this fed state. The fed state is when your body is in the process of absorbing the food you ate, digesting it and breaking it down. One of the primary reasons it is so difficult for people to lose weight while in the fed state is thanks to the high levels of insulin results from food consumption. See, a lot of people believe that if they burn more Calories they consume in a single day, they will eventually begin deriving energy from the fats stored in their body. Unfortunately, it isn't that easy. So long as your insulin levels are high, which comes from being in a fed state, your body is being signaled to burn the energy that is being taken in, not stored. It is not possible for you to burn the food you are eating, and the fact you have stored, at the same time. And if you are eating three meals a day, your body always has insulin inhibiting your stored fats from being burned. Unless you are consuming pure fat, which is very difficult and not very nutritional. The fed states will start the moment the first bite of food begins being digested, and lasts anywhere from three to five hours, depending on how much you eat and how complex it is to break down. So, even while dieting, you're going to be primarily burning the energy you've put into it. The hope is that through dieting and exercise, you'll turn the fat already stored into muscle, and what you are consuming will fuel the maintenance of that muscle.

That isn't always the case unless you're in the gym constantly.

Most diets and nutritional advice speak of how you should avoid eating a large meal before you sleep. In fact, if you are dieting, your best bet is to eat three to five hours before rest. And here's the big secret. You're already fasting if you do that. Each night, your body begins to pull the nutrients from your stored fats, since your insulin levels are now low enough to permit this. That's why you burn Calories in your sleep. However, most people don't follow this. The average individual eats dinner anywhere from 7:30 pm to 9 pm, according to a study on American dietary habits. If you take this into account, coupled with the fact that most people don't just eat three meals a day, but three meals a day plus sugary drinks and small snacks, explains a lot. It's is a big answer to why stored fat builds up so fast, even when counting Calories. On your average western diet, you're never burning what's stored. Yet, if you fast for just 24 hours, taking in only water, your body switches gears. It knows that just like when you are sleeping, you aren't taking any Calories in for fuel. And that's why your body has fat in the first place. To sustain you over periods of time like that. It'll take the average 2,000 Calories needed to sustain you through the day and burn about half a pound of fat to do it. Back in the early days, when we were still hunters and gatherers, humans couldn't eat all the time. They had to search for food. And just like when they were sleeping, the body needed some method of propelling it forward during the hunt or the gathering. That is where this process came from. Fasting isn't really some unnatural or unhealthy method of weight loss if done right. In fact, your body was pretty much designed for it. Designed to burn fats after periods of not eating. You're simply taking advantage of a very intuitive and organic process. It'd be happening anyway if we didn't live in a land of excess where we have been conditioned to constantly consume.

Your body isn't dumb. The human body is an intricate "machine" that's designed survival methods over thousands of years of evolution. None of us have lived for a thousand years and very few of us are smarter than the intelligent design of our body. It's not going to waste good fat that can "save your life" in a dire situation. It's going to let you use what you're putting in and hold onto the excess for a future emergency. Who knows when you'll be trapped in the woods without food for days? Hopefully never. Still, what if you get sick? Your body knows these things can happen, and it'd rather we "hold onto a few pounds" than let us die. And in most cases, that's great. Except we're always eating, and most of the time we are eating more than we need. But what about the conventional diet advice? You know, that method that says eat six times a day and you'll reduce Calories and fat? Well, it doesn't really matter what you are eating, or how small it is. If it is providing your body with insulin, you're forcing your system to take the energy you needed from that lowered Calorie intake, and not stored fats. You'll lose a little fat as first, but your body's smart. It's going to adapt. Sooner rather than later, you won't build up fat and you won't lose it either. Worse yet, you're going to suffer from a lack of nutrition. You'll feel cold, hungry, and tired as your metabolism and body functions shut down. And while you're suffering, you're gaining nothing. Your weight loss has stopped, and you're ready to call it quits.

This is when so many people say, "enough dieting" and pick up the health practice of fasting. Some quick research shows it is been done for thousands of years. It's easy to debunk the myth that fasting doesn't work when losing the way. And with all those additional health benefits we discussed earlier, it's just a no brainer. Your body was designed to fast, and it doesn't want you eating constantly. It wants a healthy balance between the states of fasting and fed. Enough eating to gain the necessary nutrients require for life, and enough fasting to pull additional nutrients from that excess fat build up that comes from out of whack eating habits.

This is how fasts like the juice fast and liquid fast are anything but. You're not sending your body into a state of fasting. You're just taking in all those Calories through a different process. And while your body may process them faster, it'll adapt. And eventually, the weight loss will stop, just like any other diet. A lot of people gain weight, rather than lose it, taking in unexpected excess Calories through these faux fasts. This may be why the practice of intermittent fasting is taking the world by storm. Not only is it a true fast, but it's simpler than dieting and yields more benefits. If done right, you can increase your weight loss results radically.

Let's compare some reported results of weight loss through these different fasts, and how they measure up against the intermittent fast. We'll begin with the juice fast. For this, we'll call on Mister Hypothetical again. Remembering his BMR (Basal Metabolic Rate) was 1,600, and assuming he lives a sedentary life like most of us, we'll say he burns 2,000 Calories a day. Taking on the adventure of the juice fast, Mister Hypothetical juices to have one fruit juice a day, one veggie juice a day, and two smoothies a day. It's important to note that these are very conservative estimates. Most people on the juice fast are drinking smoothies and are drinking them anywhere from three to four times a day. Why? Because they sate those "hunger pains" that juices typically don't. But let's keep Mister Hypothetical conservative. Your average tall glass of juice is approximately 224 Calories. Your average glass of veggie juice is 208 Calories. Depending on where Hypothetical is getting his smoothies from, they'll anywhere from 326 Calories to 496 Calories. That's a whopping 1,254 Calories a day. We know it takes 3,500

Calories to burn off a pound of fat, from when Mister Hypothetical was trying his hand at dieting. His caloric deficit on an average day of the juice fast is 746 Calories and observing this fast for seven days in a row yields a haughty 5,222 Calories burnt off in a week. Of course, we discussed how your body won't burn stored fat when it's getting food. Mister Hypothetical is burning off somewhere around a pound and a half in that week, but it's coming from a loss of muscle mass and water weight. His fat percentage remains untouched at the end of this fast.

Now, how about water fast? Say Mister Hypothetical observes it for one week, which is ill-advised. He's consuming zero Calories a day though, and that means 2,000 Calories are being consumed from fat stores each day. He's losing about four pounds this week, though one to two of that will come from excess waste and water being pushed through the body. Unfortunately, when you go from not eating anything to eating like you used to, your metabolism gets very confused. It thinks you're wandering without food and starts storing fats at a higher rate than before. This is the primary reason that the water fast is only advised for a day to three days. Not to mention you're trying to perform all your daily activities of going to and from work for a whole week without putting anything in your body.

Say we try out the liquid fast next. Mister Hypothetical missed his coffee on the juice fast, so he thinks this is a better alternative. The average person puts two tablespoons of sugar and one ounce of half and a half in a single cup of coffee and drinks about two to three cups a day. But Mister Hypothetical is fasting and is using coffee as a big part of filler since he read it helps with hunger management. His cup of coffee with two tablespoons of sugar and an ounce of half and half is 137 Calories. That's 548 Calories in a day. Hypothetical also drink two protein shakes a day, each at 269 Calories, plus a smoothie at lunch, 326 Calories. On this liquid diet, Mister Hypothetical is consuming 1,412 Calories a day, leaving his caloric deficit at 588, and giving him 4,116 Calories. This is a little over one pound of weight loss. But he's not losing fat, and that's because his body never got to actually fast. What's been shed is realistically just lean muscle mass and water weight.

And how does Mister Hypothetical like intermittent fasting? Let's go back our example back in Chapter 1. Our friend here was eating grapes when he got to work, 67 Calories, an egg sandwich at lunch, 390 Calories, and a milkshake with 350 Calories at the end of his eight-hour feasting period. That's only 807 Calories in a day. Now, we could stop there, but I want you to get a full perspective on how great intermittent fasting is when compared to other fasts. Say Mister Hypothetical brought a chicken sandwich home and eats that in the office at the beginning of his fast. That's an additional 200 calories, leaving him at 1,007 Calories in the day. The caloric deficit total is 993, and he's burning 6,951 Calories a day. That's two pounds a week. And because his body is in a fasting state for 16 hours out of the day? That's being burnt from fat stores, not just from the Calories he's consuming. Meaning he's getting thinner, and not just losing muscle mass. That's while eating real foods, and not worrying about his diet. No more protein shakes for you, Mister Hypothetical.

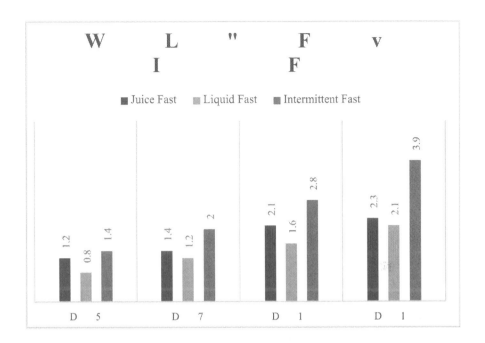

What's the final verdict? Well, when on a classic "fast" like the ones mentioned earlier, you're cutting your Calories alright. But you're rarely hitting that goal of getting your body to fast, and that means you're not likely to lose much weight. On top of this, nobody can drink fruit smoothies and protein shakes forever. Not only would you despise it, but your body will adapt. It's just not a realistic way of keeping the weight off, especially with the excess sugars you'll be consuming. And of course, you can't survive off water your whole life. The liquid fast had our hypothetical man burning 4,116 Calories a week. On the juice fast, he shed about 5,222 Calories. While water fasting for a week, he obliterated 14,000 Calories. But intermittent fasting helped burn 6,951 Calories, and most of the weight loss was actual fat! Instead of losing his hard-earned muscle mass, and feeling week constantly, Mister Hypothetical is shedding actual fat pounds and in a feasible manner. There is no starving himself on pure liquids, low energy levels, or disruption to his metabolism. The icing on the cake? He can continue this weight loss method for as long as he wants and avoid the suffering that comes from more radical fasts. While other fasting methods may just be "fads", you can see how Intermittent Fasting can be considered a real option if you want to lose weight without much sacrifice! With greater results, no less.

Chapter 4: Why Intermittent Fasting?

We've gone over the history of intermittent fasting. Seeing how it's been used to help extend the life and sharpen the mind for thousands of years. We've covered how absolutely amazing the results of fasting are when held up against the dieting. Enough to certainly make us question why they are spoken of as "fad diets" when a fast isn't a diet at all. There is no wonder that it wasn't just ancient geniuses who used this process, but also modern icons as well. Celebrities love intermittent fasting, and by looking at the weight loss provided, that's no surprise. In fact, they've always loved the intermittent fast and partial fast. When we investigate deeper, we see how intermittent fasting possesses a remarkable ability to target stored fats directly. This unique trait is not found among any other diet or weight loss method around, or at least none that can achieve it so easily. It's a process that's been honed and developed through thousands of years of the human body's evolution. Not only is it natural, but it's also incredibly good for us. And it has only been over the course of centuries that overconsumption has set up this illusion. It almost as if we've lost sight of this ability hidden within us. This amazing process that was given to us through years of logical choices the keep strongest, and the fittest, alive. Yet, thanks to so many misleading practices and restrictive views of westernized medicine, fasting has gained a not so popular reputation. One that's being thrown away, granted. However, this reputation is based solely on the "fad diets" and "faux fasting" we discussed in the last chapter. And now we see the truth.

Despite all of this "unpopular opinion", intermittent fasting still gathers attention and popularity around the world. It always has. And then the research from across seas became public. Mystifying results, the revelations that these tests and studies yielded were just too impressive to overlook. If all of this was the real deal or even half of it, then what we knew about fasting was all wrong. What we didn't know, or what the rumors kept us from knowing, was the reality. With this taking place, it was decided that we need to educate ourselves and try it out. Rather than trust conflicting studies alone, we needed to come to our own conclusions. The ballots were casts, the votes came in, and the consensus was that it was all true. It was just these faux fasts that spread unpopular opinion and misinformation.

When it comes to other methods of fasting, very few of them come close to delivering the results found through intermittent fasting. Even when these other forms of fasting provide the weight loss promised, it takes a ton out of you. Could you imagine spending a whole week on the water fast, or 21 days on the Daniel fast? Perhaps the more daring of you can! And there's nothing wrong with that. In fact, you should pat yourself on the back for having a desire to investigate this health practice. But even when someone gets past the fast itself, we see how it can so often be for nothing. Either the results are fleeting, or illusionary. Perhaps they'll lose weight by shedding water or abandoning the muscle mass they once had, but their fat will remain. And what's worse, it can play games with the metabolism. When all is said and done, someone doing the juice fast or liquid fast is probably going to end up putting on weight faster, unless the person fasting would like to keep starving themselves through liquids or water. This must be why results have shown intermittent fasting to be the most reliable method.

Intermittent fasting first gained attention from scientists in 1945, when its effects were studied on mice in a lab. This was the research we mentioned back in Chapter 2. Intermittent fasting didn't disappear after that though. It was consistently studied and made a common health practice in European countries like Germany, where plenty of discoveries on fasting have come from. Of course, when celebrities began to hear of the phenomenal claims coming from research, there was a natural level of intrigue. Hollywood always desired to be on the cutting edge of weight loss and health practices. Traveling across seas, they picked up the habit to help balance their lifestyle and weight. When the celebrities weren't the ones traveling, it was the nutritionists and fitness trainers. However, for at least half a century, intermittent fasting was a well-kept secret amongst people who lived in Europe, scientists, and the celebrity socialites that could travel between. It wasn't that the method didn't work, it was just that nutritionists on our side of the sea have refuted eating anything less than three square meals a day since the time we were able to acquire such monumental portions of food on a daily basis. Remember, it wasn't always this way when we had to provide for ourselves. Yet, in the other countries, where food was scarce or diets were different, eating at only certain points in the day was completely common. Or maybe the average person simply disliked the idea of going hungry at any point in time. It's only natural. It has only been within the last few decades that personal healthcare and self-education on these matters became popular in our culture.

To be blunt, western concepts on nutrition and healthcare have always put a big hush on fasting, intermittent or otherwise. Overconsumption not only keeps the market for food running high, making many people fat with wealth, it also keeps the medical industry well supplied with unhealthy individuals needing their care. Is this such a surprise? Countless medical problems that have plagued Americans for years have risen as effects of overconsumption. And we saw, through the studies referenced earlier, that numerous diseases that western medicine treats through elaborate methods can be more efficiently combated, and even prevented, through simply letting your body do what it has been designed to. Excess sugar intake can compromise your immune system, and lead to an increased risk of obesity, diabetes, and heart diseases. A report shows that 90% of Americans do not receive enough chromium from their diet thanks to excess consumption of refined starches. And if you are wondering why chromium is important, it is an essential mineral that is needed within the human body. It is only required in trace amounts, yet it improves insulin sensitivity, as well as augmenting protein, carbohydrate, and lipid metabolism. Taking it a step further, we know excess sugar consumption can be linked to loosened skin and premature aging, thanks to its power to rob your proteins of their normal ability to keep your skin elastic. To top it off, sugar has been found to affect the parts of your brain that control cognition, even inhibiting their development in children. Certain types of diabetes have been connected to unneeded consumption of carbohydrates (NIDDM). And a number of cancers have been linked to excessive carbohydrate intake from refined sources, as well as a few gastrointestinal diseases. We're starting to see a pattern, right? Even a high-fat diet has been linked to a plethora of chronic diseases, namely heart diseases and cancers. As you can see, the two largest killers we are facing today are results of overconsumption.

We're getting better though. Intermittent fasting didn't regain popularity and attention with the public until 2012. The first wave of interest sprouted from the United Kingdom, when BBC2 released a televised documentary on Horizon. This documentary was called *Eat, Fast and Live Longer*, and sparked a high demand for information in the community. It highlighted the benefits and debate over fasting while elaborating on how helpful intermittent fasting has always been in natural healthcare. The documentary cultured a notable amount of curiosity in the 5:2 fasting method while opening a new wave of dialogue. Research and reports suddenly began to be released, new and old, supporting the science behind fasting. Many of these were published in best-selling books that took the UK by storm.

Not too much farther down the line, intermittent fasting became a popular health care practice. It is believed that Silicon Valley companies were some of the first to start advocating the weight loss method, hoping to gain a reputation of compassion and concern over the health of their employees. They were aiming to create a trend of happiness, and it worked for some time. We all know how the world looks to Silicon Valley and the tech industry. Knowing this, it isn't hard to imagine how people heard far and wide about this practice sweeping the "innovative and progressive" tech center of the world. From there it wasn't long that all the celebrities came out announcing they've been using the intermittent fast for years. They couldn't have told us a little sooner? And the story goes on, and so on, as the wave passed through communities. It spread into Canada; the seal was broken! By then, the wide range of information on the internet was at our fingertips and people were able to cut through the veil of misinformation surrounding fasting. It is important to note that fasting has been misused and abused through history as well though. As we discussed, there have been plenty of "faux fasts" that are just diets marketing themselves under new names. Not only that but when the 5:2 method of fasting became popular, the false belief spread that you can eat literally "any junk under the sun". So long as you fast two days a week. This is not true. Remember the golden rule, avoid carbs at all costs. And keep in mind that nearly all the health benefits we find linked to intermittent fasting are a result of avoiding over-consumption. So, if you're not eating for two days of the week, and then eating four cheeseburgers a week, your health is still going to suffer. A feast day isn't an excuse to binge on unhealthy fast foods. Of course, this doesn't mean that the 5:2 fast isn't reliable for achieving improved health. It just means that it has been done right. Don't worry though! That's why materials like this book exist. To make sure you cut through the misinformation and use the intermittent fasting method that will be best for you.

Seeing how intermittent fasting is just about the only viable option for fasting in general, do we really have to question the "why" so much? If all that "mind-bending" research in Chapter 2 didn't eliminate any uncertainty that fasting is great for your health and will give you more results than you've bargained for, then don't fret. Those were only the most radical of health benefits, and there are so many more. We haven't covered how intermittent fasting truly affects your metabolism and the science behind it. How adrenaline levels rise, growth hormone increases, and it can turn your metabolism into a more efficient means of making muscle. The facts are that fasting augments your health. And it will cleanse your system of a variety of factors that normally inhibit weight loss. One such aid to your metabolic state is the benefit of a reduction in insulin levels. If you remember our explanation between the fasted state and the fed state from the last chapter, you'll recognize the importance of insulin. If you don't, no need to worry. You don't need to know why it's important to actually benefit from the reduction of insulin in your bloodstream. And you don't need to how it works just too fast. The ancients had no idea, but that didn't stop them from encouraging it, even amongst students. Still, let's take a moment to explain it further. Insulin plays a monumental role in dictating whether you are burning stored fats or the Calories absorbed through foods you eat. It is one of the primary factors in deciding whether you are "fasting" or "fed". But why does this happen? Or rather, how?

Well, in scientific terms, we say that insulin inhibits lipolysis and gluconeogenesis. It is a common fact in physiology, but not common for the people being told to eat three meals a day. So, what is lipolysis exactly? And why does it matter? Well, lipolysis is discussed fairly often among biologists. It is defined as the process through which the fats in our bodies are eliminated, broken down, or removed. Simply put, it takes the fat you've stored and makes it into available energy. This is typically done through the enzymes in our bodies, as well as water and hydrolysis. When glucose levels in the human body are found lacking or running low, lipolysis begins. This happens most often between meals, or on a fast! Lipolysis then helps loosen up those stored fats, converting them into something we can use. It makes them flow freely through the bloodstream in the form of "fatty acids", which then can be broken down by the metabolism to fuel the body, being forged into potential energy in the absence of consumed nutrients. This process is vital to other functions of the body as well, like gluconeogenesis and cellular respiration! In short, lipolysis is an essential function in the body that helps sustain life. And through over-consumption of foods, raising insulin levels, we prevent this process from taking place. This is just one-way fasting helps maintain proper metabolic health.

And gluconeogenesis? For those of you that are wondering what in the world that is, biology defines this function as the process of the body allowing new glucose molecules to be formed rather than being produced through a molecular deconstruction of glycogen. It's your body making sure you can survive when you aren't eating. A biological mechanism that takes place in the liver, and sometimes in the kidney and small intestine. But why does this matter? How is it important? Well, glucose is a vital factor in producing the energy molecule adenosine triphosphate. Some people worry that when they stop eating, they will lose energy. Yet, this molecular process was evolved to address that very barrier. What happens is, when your body can't create glucose nutrients being digested, gluconeogenesis occurs. This way, in times of fasting, you can still receive proper energy from glucose being produced in your body, without having to worry about insulin levels getting in your way. Through this factor, you can burn your stored fats, and still hit the gym or go through your day-to-day office routine. Whichever you prefer.

What else can affect metabolism? We know our bodies are very intricate, and that there are many different factors that can influence this process. A healthy metabolism is very important to more than just weight, so the more we know about it, the better. One scientific research article, labeled "Metabolic Effects of Intermittent Fasting", compiles data of several studies into one comprehensive read, though there are no explanations translated into layman's terms. However, within this article, they discuss intermittent fasting's effects on the circadian rhythm within our bodies. If you do not know what the circadian rhythm is, I'll break it down. Over time, living creatures have evolved to follow patterns of day and night. It is based on the 24-hour light and dark cycles that take place on this planet. Essentially, this clock keeps our behavioral patterns, our activity patterns, and our body's internal processes, all in check. It helps limit activity at night and increases productivity during the day. The circadian rhythm helps tell our body how to function, and when to have our metabolism perform certain functions. Functions that we would like to be performed more often, like burning fat stored or producing extra adrenaline. There is also science to show that this "clock" helps control certain functions within the liver, fat, and skeletal muscle cells. A massive trigger for this process is when your body is in a state of feeding or in a state of fasting. The working theory of this article is that, within a normal three meal a day diet, we interrupt the natural functions triggered by the circadian rhythm. Based on the research the authors have gathered, it is observed that eating out of the natural evolutionary pattern results in disrupting processes that are essential to strong metabolic health. Not only that, but these feeding patterns have also been linked to increased risks of cardiometabolic diseases and cancers. The pattern shows itself again.

Some of the impacts our circadian rhythm has on metabolism determine factors like insulin sensitivity, which is noted to decrease through the day and into the night. Why is this important? Because insulin sensitivity determines how long it takes for your body to begin making use of fats stored within it. However, this only takes place during a time period when your body believes you are not eating. Likewise, when you eat at night, glucose responses to meals are notably heightened. So, you begin storing fats rather than eating them. This is associated with late afternoon meals, like dinners and midnight snacks. This takes place thanks to growth hormones and insulin inhibitors being released within the body to allow your metabolic system to switch gears. Meaning, when your body should be normally turning fat into energy, eating three meals a day will compromise this process. Studies have shown that this cycle can be naturally extended by simply eating later in the day, rather than when you first wake. This will increase the amount of energy being taken from fat stores so that you are burning it continuously thanks to your fasted state and the circadian rhythm. This is the basis for intermittent fasting and using this evolutionary function to kick your metabolism into overdrive.

Fasting has also been linked to an increase in epinephrine and norepinephrine, better known as adrenaline and noradrenaline. Like what was discussed earlier, the theory is that this is connected to an extension of the circadian rhythm. As we know, when the body enters the fasted state through lowered insulin, it begins to release certain circadian triggers. When the body enters the night cycle of the circadian, it helps regulate the metabolic system to preserve us while we rest. Likewise, as an adaptation of humans over thousands of years, it is triggered prematurely during intermittent or extended fasts. As we have discussed, this is a significant theory in how the body prevents so many different illness and diseases through fasting. Epinephrine and norepinephrine levels help keep our energy high, our metabolism working a top capacity, and play several other roles in both the mind and body, like fueling the immune system. Those with epinephrine and norepinephrine deficiencies experience increased levels of anxiety and depression, fibromyalgia, hypoglycemia, migraines, sleep disorders, and the dreaded restless leg syndrome. Of course, more adrenaline will also help you a few other ways, giving you that extra boost you may need to be active. In fact, this is another reason we find ourselves even more energetic while fasting. Your body is pumping you full of more adrenaline, to see you through to your next meal! And if you are looking to build muscle while on a fast, this will be one of many gifts your body provides. Another gift is the extra growth hormones that will be released.

We all know that Growth Hormone, or GH, is extremely important. You don't need to be a scientist to tell what it is used for since its right there in the name. However, there has been an increased interest in stimulating growth hormone through many different methods. Some people believe that by injecting HGH, Human Growth Hormone, they can reverse aging and increase physical performance. Primarily, we see this in the ring of top tier athletes and competitors. We've already seen how fasting slows the aging process. There are certain theories that link this to an increase in Growth Hormone. GH is a microscopic protein that is formed and released to help physical development; this takes place through the pituitary gland. Once it is made, the hormone floods into the bloodstream, sent into the liver, which stimulates the production of IGF-1, a mediator in the communication with your body. This then travels through the various organs and cells. It shouts commands, telling you to grow, grow and grow some more. IGF-1 promotes cellular development in cells, while growth hormone stimulates other parts of the body. But what parts of you are going to see the greatest benefits from this? Your kidneys, your liver, bones, muscles and cartilage, and even the nerves of your skin! In adults, it helps keep body composition regular, encourages healthy muscle and bone growth, aids in metabolism processes like burning fats and sugars, and may even be key in keeping the heart muscles healthy. Growth Hormone is released rather erratically in us as we grow older. Exercise is one way to trigger this release, but research on the effects of intermittent fasting and GH have revealed something that the athletes out there may be pleased to know. The title of one scientific study says it all. "Fasting Enhances Growth Hormone Secretions and Amplifies the Complex Rhythms of Growth Hormone Secretion", that's a mouthful. Yet, it is a great thing to know. The study links the increased duration of the circadian rhythm while on a fast to the increased secretion of Growth Hormones in individuals fasting. This is supported by the fact that the body releases most Growth Hormone secretions during the night. "Through our research, we found that a restricted calorie intake achieved through alternate or intermittent fasting is a deciding factor for increased release of GH secretion from the penial gland." Could this be one of the many reasons extreme athletes participate in intermittent and partial fasting, like the One Meal a Day method?

We mentioned Keto earlier. A reason that fasting is truly amazing is that you can send your body into ketosis, without the rigorous dieting practices. We know the results you desire from an intermittent fast are weight loss. Yes, all these radical health benefits, whether it's the release of Growth Hormone, Autophagy, or a more efficient metabolism, are not the true point of why you chose this book. We know what you really want. To get rid of your fat, in the most natural method possible. This is a process that both Intermittent Fasting and the Keto diet have in common. Though only the intermittent fast can achieve it so simply. Burning fat, instead of Calories. With Keto you will have to eat a very exclusive diet, avoiding all carbs, sugars, and preventing insulin levels from rising. Once insulin has dropped low enough, ketosis begins. However, through intermittent fasting, you can send your body into ketosis without any hassle, and without dodging foods. It may take longer, but the process will happen repeatedly once you are on your intermittent fast for a week or so. You can aid in this by avoiding carbs in your diet on your feast days, or in the periods that you are eating. Unlike fasting, Keto does not guarantee to burn fat straight from your stores. Instead, you'll have to burn through the fat and protein you've eaten during the day and hope you didn't consume some hidden sugars or carbs. Fasting will cut out the middle man as we said. By sticking to it, you'll be burning off your fat and even reaching ketosis without the diet, if you so desire.

When all is said and done, your body isn't going to degrade or break down, as the rumors say. Scientific data has uncovered the exact opposite. In fact, one of the best methods to build up lean muscle mass is through the intermittent fast. This is a big inverse from dieting that almost always forces your body to be malnourished, which stops muscles from getting the necessary nutrients. The results of fasting done right will take advantage of the release of growth hormones and testosterone to fuel your body and your workouts, helping you reach new goals and tackle the most difficult sections of fat. The results speak for themselves. When you're fasting and feeding, what happens is your body produces more uncoupling proteins. And what those proteins do is they poke holes in the mitochondria. Anyone who's taken high school biology knows that mitochondria are the powerhouse of the cell, they turn what we eat into ATP or adenosine triphosphate. So, what happens is, the mitochondria composition changes so that you're producing less energy and more heat. You're burning more calories just sitting. But when it comes to building muscle, the meal after your fast is what becomes even more important for muscle growth. A high protein meal will give the uncoupling proteins an even greater rise. And this is when you train when you're in your feeding period. Because what will happen is your body will take that protein and use it even more efficiently, breaking it down almost immediately and turning it into pure gains. "It was pretty surprising. When I first fasted, I thought I was going to lose it all. Fat, yeah. But muscle too. How can my muscles get the proper nutrients when I'm not feeding them? I didn't realize that instead of ignoring my fat, it was going to use those stores to feed my body. Including my muscles. And somehow, I last longer in the gym, and my growth reflects that. My body fat is down by at least 3%, I was originally at 14%. I've been able to beat more than a few personal bests in the gym in the year I've been using the intermittent fast. And my muscle mass has gone up ten pounds. I've got more energy to burn, way more adrenaline. I'm happier, I'm leaner, and I'm stronger. I've only been to the gym half the time. It's amazing."

Chapter 5: The Best Way to Begin Your Intermittent Fast

Congratulations on making it this far! I know, we've come a long way. I'm sure you feel like an absolute expert on fasting by now. No doubt about it, you may even feel ready to go give a lecture on the subject. And with all the information you've gained, you really might be. That was certainly the goal, at the very least! To provide you with enough research, explanation, and detail to truly depict how powerful intermittent fasting is as a health practice, not mention a tool for weight loss. To lend you every bit of information available on the internet that might make you feel more comfortable with the concept of fasting, and even get you excited about it. With all the potential health benefits that you'll receive through this practice, you're certainly not going to regret. And if you've made it this far, I know without a doubt that you are ready to begin your fast. Within this chapter, I will do my absolute best to list every single tip, trick, and method that may make your fasting process as simple as possible.

By now, the concept of fasting shouldn't intimidate you. You've seen how it has been used throughout the ages. One would argue that the wisest individuals in history have used fasting to expand their minds and extend their lives. And through the last few chapters, you've steadily learned how deep the scientific research runs. The evidence supporting fasting, especially intermittent fasting, as a great method of weight loss and health care, is substantial. There should be no remnant of doubt or skepticism in your mind. If you're hoping to lose weight in a process that is simpler, you were right to read this book. You can lose weight, you can live a healthier life, and you can do it all through a natural method that will be as easy as eating your breakfast later in the day and your dinner earlier. So, my hope is that the only thing you might be feeling, that isn't excitement or curiosity, is overwhelmed. By all the answers, all the knowledge, and all the potential ways to fast.

Yes, there are a lot of different fasting methods out there. A lot of practices that can all give you efficient weight loss through simplistic practices. So, the first suggestion I can give you on how to begin your fast is this. Just try it. Don't worry about all the different types of fasting just yet. Start small. You know the science, so you know that even half a day of drinking only water will give you an idea of what fasting is like. The real trick is reassuring yourself that it is no loss. And based all the benefits that come from intermittent fasting, it won't be a loss. In fact, if you have any experience with dieting in the first place, this is going to be even easier. Because, instead of having to go out and buy certain foods, or plan how or where you can eat, you just have to pick a time where you won't eat. Do you like your breakfast? You can fast through the middle of the day, just for a few hours, to get a feel for the process. What the hunger will be like, and what going through the day without food is like. The biggest thing you'll notice is that you'll have more time on your hands. So, try to fill it with something productive. It's almost like when someone quits smoking. They say that once you get past the oral fixation, the biggest challenge is finding out how to replace the time you used to spend on smoke breaks. It's the same concept. As a consumer culture, we don't realize just how much time we spend eating. Or how often we are eating when we aren't actually hungry. Sometimes, people just eat to do something they feel is productive. With the time you'll suddenly find on your hands, you can do a lot. You can read a favorite book, study a new language, and research something that you're curious about, or even take care of personal chores. Either way, you'll find yourself feeling a bit lost when you're not cooking at your normal hour or eating on your normal lunch break. Just take advantage of that time and do something fun.

Don't try to fast a whole week straight out of the gate. If you've never fasted before, it can be a strange transition for your body. Your best bet is to gradually get your stomach used to this feeling. Start with a half a day, once a week. Once you feel like you can take on more than that, you can bump any way you see fit. If you want to fast half the day, two times a week, try it. Or maybe you want to experience a whole day of water fasting? It won't hurt you, and you'll find it easier to stand by the commitment if you know you experience a normal day of eating tomorrow. From one day a week to two days, to three days. You can work your way gradually towards fasting half a day, every day of the week! Take it as far as you want. This is your body and you know it best. The biggest advice any fitness coach or nutritionist will give you is "Pick a lane and stick to it." Teach your body to be consistent, and pick something you feel you can commit to. Once you've experienced fasting for at least four weeks in a row, I'm sure you'll have an idea of how simple it really is. From there, you can play around with all the different types of fasts.

Now to go over some of these fasting techniques for you. I'm sure you've noticed from the past couple of chapters that fasting comes in a wide variety of forms. So long as you are allowing your body the time between meals to go into a "fasting" state, you're in the green. Remember, it takes your body three to five hours since your last meal to stop digesting and begin fasting. The easiest method to start with is the "12 hour" fast, which was the one I mentioned above. It's as simple as the name implies. You block a portion of 12 hours that you won't take in any Calories, and all you will drink is water. This is by far the easiest method to begin, because you may already be fasting in this way as we speak. Most fasts incorporate the time you sleep into the schedule. The best way to give this a shot is fasting from 7 p.m. to 7 a.m. so that you are still about to eat breakfast. The reason we choose 7 p.m. is that it will take your body a minimum of three hours to enter the fasted state and resting going to sleep while your body is digesting will inhibit the fat loss process that comes through fasting. If you believe you can get your dinner in earlier, that's great. As a rule of thumb, you should always try to eat dinner as early as possible.

Once you've gotten the hang of the "12-hour" fast, maybe trying it for a couple over the span of a few weeks, you're welcome to try out the 5:2 method. You're going to want to choose two days out of the week, preferably separate, and fast on them. This will be a whole day fast, where you consume below 500 to 600 Calories. Now, if you haven't taken a whack at a whole day fast yet, you might want to try it before attempting this 5:2 method. It really isn't all that scary, however. If you've gone a whole day without eating, the two days you will be fasting would be nothing in comparison. Mainly because, on those fast days, you're still allowed those 500 to 600 Calories. That can be two sandwiches if you keep them lean. The important thing to keep in mind is consistency. Your metabolism is going to help you shed the fat, but if you stop fasting and start overeating with three square meals a day, the weight can come right back on. It's important to note that on your five feasting days, you're eating healthy and with the normal Calorie count. If you try "making up" for the days you fasted, your metabolism will get confused. Another important trick to the 5:2 method is switching the two days each week. Your body is intelligent and intuitive. If you stay too consistent, it will adapt and start holding onto weight to make up for the fast days. Always keep one feast day between your fast days and do your best to rotate and change them up.

A quick side note for you. If you're experiencing hunger pains or just hunger in general, try a cup of plain black coffee. The Calorie count is practically non-existent, which means it won't bring your body out of the fasting state. The beverage has been linked to a reduction in the hormones that tell your body you are hungry and may reduce the bacteria within the gut that creates that hunger sensation. On top of this helpful effect, caffeine has been shown to stimulate neurological pathways and aid in the metabolic burn. This specifically takes place when high quantities of raw caffeine enter the bloodstream, such as with a strong cup of black coffee.

Teas are also good for this as well, such as green tea, though make sure to watch your Calorie count. Another helpful not, do not consume zero calorie sodas or anything of the like. There has been researching showing that, even though the sweeteners are zero calories, they trick your brain and body into thinking you're eating real sugar, which can force it out of the fasting state. Better safe than sorry.

Another type of intermittent fasting is the Alternate Day fast. This is an extended version of the 5:2 fast where, instead of fasting for only two days out of the week, you fast every other day in the week. You can start with a fast day on Sunday, or a fast day on Monday, whichever you prefer. Results for this can vary, depending on your method. Some people choose to consume 500 – 600 Calories on their fast days, while others drink strictly water for the whole day. The truly important part is, just like with the 5:2 method, not over-consuming on your feast days. Your appetite should naturally decrease over time, but you can easily get caught up in overeating because you "think you need it". And remember, just because you're fasting doesn't mean you should pump your body full of sugars or greasy fast food. Eating healthy should always be a goal, but you don't have to follow any specific diet to lose weight while fasting. So long as you are balancing the methods. Whether it's low-calorie consumption or absolute fasting on your Alternate Day fast, it's going to be quite intense at first. So, make sure to work towards this method at your own pace.

If the idea of fasting every other day doesn't strike your fancy, there are plenty of other ways to do it. There is the weekly 24-hour fast, for one. Also, known as a water fast, it's selecting one day out of the week where you will eat nothing and drink only water. However, you practice this method at least once a week, though some people do it twice. On this fast, you can have water, coffee, and tea. Make sure to avoid those artificial sweeteners I mentioned earlier that they can still trick your brain into believing you are off your fast. This is very important to remember because a lot of fasting advice out there labels "Zero Calorie" drinks as okay. However, if they contain those artificial sweeteners, they are anything but. Unsweetened iced tea and drinks like that are no problem though. When going back to your regular eating habits, be sure to avoid overeating, and do your best to eat things that will only feed your body the best nutrients. While this isn't a necessary part of the fast, eating nothing but carbs the next day or eating double your normal Calorie intake can delay or negate the effects of fasting.

Some of you out there may have heard of the OMAD diet, though this is a misnomer. OMAD is fast, and it stands for "One Meal a Day". This practice focuses on allowing your body to be in a fasting state for as long as possible, while still getting to eat. Typically, individuals will fast for a minimum of 23 hours a day. However, there are a few approaches to eating a single meal a day. Some people suggest eating one meal at night is the best method. This is not true, as we have seen how important it is for your body to begin the circadian rhythm at night. If your boy has high insulin levels while you are sleeping, not only will the night cycle not begin. The food you've eaten with will be converted into fat at an increased rate than during the day. The best method of One Meal a Day fasting around is eating the meal either a few hours after your wake, around 8 or 9 am, or eating it in the middle of the day. This will give you more time fasting effectively. Sleep is probably when you can get the easiest period of fasting in since it's when you fast naturally and when you feel the effects the least, so always try to time it into your fast.

Last, but not least, there is the 16:8 method. This is probably the easiest to maintain, and you can follow the method every day if you like. You just fast for 16 hours, and then eat within an 8-hour window. You can achieve this relatively easily, and I recommend trying it out before moving onto more extreme measures of fasting, like Alternate Day fasts or One Meal a Day. This particular method is believed to yield the most benefits with the least effort. It's great for the individuals who tried the 12-hour fast and didn't see much benefit. An easy way to start is fasting from 6 p.m. the night before, until 10 a.m. the next day. The eight-hour window you can eat in would be 10 a.m. to 6 p.m., giving you a regular mid-day eating schedule. You can still have breakfast, though late, and still, eat lunch at the office. So long as you get home early enough, you can even eat dinner with the family. 16:8 is the same method used by so many celebrities, and it's yielded some of the most impressive results. It's certainly the most common fasting method out there, right next to the 5:2 method. Namely, because you can use it every day, and you may not even realize it. In fact, a lot of people are only a slight tweak away from taking part in a 16:8 fast.

Remember, while you're fasting you want to stay as hydrated as possible. Your body is going to be searching for energy, and by providing it with plenty of water you ensure that it has all it needs to keep your blood and metabolism flowing. On average, you should try to drink 2 to 3 liters of water in a day, just to maintain your body's normal functions. If you don't drink enough water on fasting days, not only can it be seriously detrimental to your health, but it can make the whole thing a real chore. If you're getting headaches, that's a good sign that you need more water. When you're getting those hunger pains, don't sit there a dwell on the turkey sandwich your co-worker is gorging on. Take the time to do something you like that will distract you from the thoughts of food. Get ahead on your paperwork or fill out a crossword. Obsessive thoughts are the biggest challenge to overcome in fasting and the number one thing that breaks the commitment. Remember, you don't need food to get the energy you need. That energy can easily be taken from your fat instead. Your body is just telling you to eat as an alert so that you know it is going to start processing fat if you don't. After a few days of fasting, the cravings will fade. In fact, you'll begin to feel better while fasting, thanks to an increase of metabolic energy and adrenaline. Some people who fast for long periods of time, or even every day, forget that they need to eat. It's because you will start to feel sluggish and weighed down when in a fed state, thanks to a rise in insulin levels. And while you can work out on a fast, it is recommended you only follow light workouts like stretches and yoga. If you're going to perform an intensive workout, try and fit it into your feasting days or periods. This way your body is getting all the necessary nutrients that you want to turn into muscle. If you're going to eat heavily on your feasting days, we recommend a minimal about of cardio or taking a walk after your meal to help digest it properly. If you're finding it hard to resist eating, you can ask yourself why you're eating in the first place. Are you upset? Are you bored? Is there something on your mind that is making you stress eat?

You've decided to lose weight by now, but how do you track that? It's important to keep in mind that your body can gain or lose weight for just about a dozen reasons. So, whether or not you are seeing progress does not necessarily mean you aren't losing fat. The important thing is to account for the fluctuations in your weight. First thing you'll need is a halfway decent body scale. Not every scale is built to the same level of precision, so make sure you read the reviews if you're going to buy one offline. Next, you'll need to weigh yourself at least twice a day. If you can fit a weigh in during the middle of the day, that's even better. However, the minimum is one weigh in in the morning, and one weigh in before you go to bed. The best way to take these measurements is naked since clothing can alter the results by a pound or more, depending on what you're wearing. Next, you're going to take the average of every weight measurement for the day. You do this by adding all your results together, then dividing them by the number of tests. Say you measure yourself twice. When you wake up in the morning, you're weighed in at 167. Then, before you go to bed, you weigh in at 165. Now you add those numbers together (167+165=332) and then you divide them by two

($332 \div 2 = 166$). If there were three tests, you'd take the three results and add them together, then divide the sum by three. To get the final results, at the end of the week you are going to take all the average you calculated, add them together, then divide them by 7, for the days in the week. Say your averages are 166, 164, 165, 164, 163, 162, and 163. ($166+164+165+164+163+162+163=1,147$) ($1,147 \div 7 = 163.857$) This means that your weekly average weight is nearly 164 pounds. Tracking this over the course of a month will show you how much weight you've lost, but we know those fluctuations can be alarming, but remember that weight doesn't directly relate to fat. You could be gaining muscle, water weight, or even the remnants of food. That is why most individuals prefer to track fat loss.

There are a lot of expensive methods that you can pay for but tracking your weight can be simple too. You don't necessarily need all the expensive equipment, especially if you are trying to lose fat from specific areas. One such method is using a body fat caliper, also known as Plicometer. You could also purchase a BIA scale or bioelectrical impedance analysis scale. This scale sends a low-level current through your body, tracking how it moves. Taking the results, it plugs in your height, weight, and gender, then calculates your body fat percentage for you. These can be costly though, and a measuring tape plus a plicometer are a fraction of the cost. So here is how to measure through skin folds. You will take the skin, fold it over and pull it away from the muscle, so there is only fat in between. The plicometer is then used to measure the thickness in millimeters, pinching the skin gently to get a gauge for the thickness. You'll want to take about two measurements, then average them. Some of the sites you can measure include the:

- Pectoral – Taken at mid-chest, just in front of the armpit
- Midaxilla – The middle of your torso, on the side
- Triceps – The back of your arm, in the upper area
- Suprailiac – Just above the hip bone, and the iliac crest
- Abdomen – Taken just to the right of the belly button
- Quadriceps – The middle of your thigh, near the upper portion

Not all measurements can be taken yourself, so you can always ask a friend or family member to help. Once this is done, take those readings and plug them into any number of online calculators, which can tell you your average body fat percentage in those areas. There are also charts that can be used as well, but I suggest you stick to online calculators since the equation is quite complex. For those of you who are curious and the DIY types, here you go:

- The Jackson and Pollock equation for Women is: 1.0994921 – (0.0009929 x the sum of the skinfold measurements in millimeters) + (0.0000023 x the sum of squared) – (0.0001392 x age)
- The Jackson and Pollock equation for Men: 1.10938 – (0.0008267 x sum) + (0.0000016 x sum squared) – (0.0002574 x age)

If you don't want to get too complex, you can also take a simple measuring tape and measure your waist occasionally, tracking how you have slimmed down during your fast. You'll want to measure just below the belly button, but not too low. The main reason this can be a confusing or unreliable method is sometimes eating and drinking can lead to bloating, depending on what you consume. If you are going to use these measurements, the rule of thumb would be to keep your timing consistent. The best bet is to measure your waist when you first wake up. You can also measure it twice a day, like with weight, and calculate the averages to give you a better idea for tracking progress. You can do this same process with other body parts as well, such as chest, thighs, and arms.

The final tool I can arm you within this weight loss adventure is Calorie counting. This will be especially important if you are planning to follow fasting methods like the Alternate Day fast or the 5:2 fast, since both of these methods call for restricting your Calorie intake to a certain amount on the fast days. Now, the best place to start with is establishing your Basic Metabolic Rate (BMR from earlier), then calculate how many calories you burn in a day with the MET key. Once you've got an idea on your average calories burned in a day, you can use this as a reference point. Say you live a mellow life or sit behind a desk all day. No worries, fasting will keep you burning that fat. Chances are that your Calorie burn in a single day is somewhere between 2,000 to 2,200. Remember caloric deficits from earlier? 500 a day to burn a pound a week. Track your Calories through nutritional labels and helpful apps, even on feasts days. That way you know how many Calories you're burning, even on the days when you aren't fasting! Feel free to go back a few chapters to remind yourself about how to create a caloric deficit. And remember, try and eat relatively healthy on your feast days. You don't have to diet, but eating healthy foods like raw fats, proteins, and veggies packed with nutrients will push your weight loss goals even further, and help you develop muscle naturally.

With these tips at your disposal, you should have no problem tracking your weight loss and sticking to your fast. I promise, once you're trying it out, you'll see that eating nothing is a lot easier than convincing yourself to eat something specific. With intermittent fasting, you don't have to dodge foods, and you don't have to worry about your Calories too much. With only so much time in the day to eat, it will be almost impossible for you to consume more Calories than you are burning in a day. Go ahead and try it out. Skip your breakfast tomorrow, and maybe even lunch if you are feeling daring. Just remember that consistency and patience will be key. With time, you'll be well adjusted and lighter than when you were eating three meals a day.

Chapter 6: How to Plan Your Fast. Recipes.

Now that you know all about the different types of fasts, I'm sure you're probably trying to form a plan on where to start. And that's not a bad idea! It's always helpful to plan ahead, like finding ways to fill the time you would have used for eating. There is more than one way to plan though! If you want to get the absolute most out of your fast, you can plan out what meals you will eat and when. Healthy meals are always the best way to go with fasting since you'll reap them most when your metabolism is in this heightened state. This way, you know for sure that you're getting every bit of nutrition you need to keep you working at maximum efficiency. Below, I will list 28 meals that can be used during an intermittent fast. They are all low in calories and provide ample amount of nutrition for your fast. There will be three per day, so that way you can use them for any fast you like.

Bite-Sized Quiche with Potato and Cheddar

Serving size for this recipe is two quiches, and it will prepare up to six. This recipe will take approximately 1 hour and 30 minutes to cook.

What's in it

377 milligrams of potassium; 494 milligrams of sodium; 2 milligrams of iron; 177 milligrams of calcium; 7 milligrams of vitamin c; 1,251 milligrams of vitamin A; 0 grams of added sugars; 3 grams of sugars; 263 milligrams of cholesterol; 14 grams of protein; 11 grams of carbohydrates; 1 gram of fiber; 16 grams of fat; for a total of 238 Calories

Ingredients:

- 1.5 c fresh spinach, chopped.5 teaspoon of black pepper, ground
- .5 c of low-fat milk
- 1 c of smoked cheddar cheese, shredded
- 8 eggs, large

- 3 quarters of a teaspoon of salt
- 1 c of red onion, diced
- 1.5 c of red-skinned potatoes, finely diced
- 2 tbsp of extra-virgin olive oil

To begin, we will need to preheat your over. The temperature you will need is 325 degrees Fahrenheit. Make sure that you have a 12-muffin tray and coat it with an oil or cooking spray.

Next, you will need a large skillet. Placing oil in, heat it over medium. This is when you will add your onions and potatoes, as well as your salt (a quarter of a teaspoon). Stir this until all is cooked through, approximately five minutes. Remove from the heat, let cool.

Time to mix your quiche. You will take your eggs, milk, peppers, and cheese, and remaining salt, mixing it into a large bowl. Make sure to add on your potato and spinach mixture, giving it a good stir. Take your quiche mixture and pour it into your muffin tin.

Time to bake! This should take approximately twenty-five minutes. Allow a cooling time of 5 minutes before popping them out of the tin.

Done!

Protein Packed Turkey Chili

Serving size is about 1 and a half c, there are approximately six servings prepared by this recipe. This should take about two hours to cook.

What's in it:

1,000 milligrams of potassium; 596 milligrams of sodium; 5 milligrams of iron; 131 milligrams of calcium; 28 milligrams of vitamin C; 216 milligrams of vitamin A; 0 grams of added sugar; 4 grams of sugar; 43 milligrams of cholesterol; 28 grams of protein; 38 grams of carbs; 10 grams of fiber; 14 grams of fat; a total of 350 Calories

Ingredients:

- 4 c of chicken broth
- 2 four oz cans of green chiles, hot or mild
- 2 15 oz cans of sodium free white beans, make sure to rinse
- .25 tsp of salt
- .5 tsp of white pepper, ground

- .5 tsp of coriander, ground
- 4 tsp of cumin, ground
- 2 tbsp of oregano, dried
- .5 c of bulgur wheat
- 2 zucchini, medium sized, diced
- 4 cloves of minced garlic
- Single onion, diced
- 1 lb of turkey, ground, 93% lean

First, you'll heat your oil over medium-high heat, with a Dutch oven. The turkey, onions, and garlic are then added. You want to break the meat up as you stir and cook, make sure that it is no longer pink. This should take three to five minutes.

After this is done, you'll stir in the zucchini and let it cook until softened. This should take five to seven minutes.

Now for the seasonings. You'll want to stir in all those ground herbs and spices, letting it cook for thirty seconds to a minute.

The chiles and beans come next, then add the broth. Let this mixture rise to a boil.

Lower the heat until the pot is simmering, stirring when needed. You'll want the liquid to boil out until the mixture is thickened and the bulgur cooked. This should take about fifty minutes.

Done!

Pancakes with Dried Blueberries and Pecans

The serving size for this recipe is 2 pancakes, and it makes 8 servings. It will take one hour to cook.

What's in it:

116 milligrams of potassium; 356 milligrams of sodium; 1 milligram of iron; 54 milligrams of calcium; 73 milligrams of vitamin A; 5 grams of added sugars; 11 grams of sugar; 47 milligrams of cholesterol; 8 grams of protein; 35 grams of carbs; 3 grams of fiber; 10 grams of fat; and a total of 255 Calories

Ingredients:
- 2 tbsp of canola oil
- 1.5 c of buttermilk, nonfat
- 2 egg whites, large
- 2 eggs, large
- .5 tsp of salt
- 1 tsp of ground cinnamon
- 2 tsp of baking powder

- 3 tablespoons of brown sugar, light
- .5 c of chopped pecans, toasted
- .5 c of blueberries, dried
- .5 c of whole-wheat flour
- 1 c of flour, all-purpose

First, we need to mix the blueberries, pecans, sugar, baking powder, cinnamon, salt, and both kinds of the flower together. Do this all in a single large bowl.

Then, you mix the oil, buttermilk, eggs, and egg whites in another bowl of medium size. In the center of the flour mixture, make a well to pour this mixture in. Stir the wet mixture and dry mixture together until the batter is smooth. A quarter cup of batter will make on the pancake.

Cook over a medium heated skilled.

Done!

Black Bean Salad

The serving size for this recipe is 2 cups and prepares 4 servings. It will take you approximately one hour to prepare.

What's in it:

1,238 milligrams of potassium; 407 milligrams of sodium; 4 milligrams of iron; 113 milligrams of calcium; 45 milligrams of vitamin C; 3,894 milligrams of vitamin A; 0 grams of added sugars; 11 grams of sugar; 0 cholesterol; 11 grams of protein; 41 grams of carbs; 13 grams of fiber; 16 grams of fat; 322 Calories in total

Ingredients:

- 1 15-oz can of black beans, be sure to rinse
- 1 pt. of halved grape tomatoes
- 2 ears of corn, or 2 cups of frozen corn, kernels separated
- 8 c of mixed greens
- .5 tsp of salt
- 1 garlic clove, minced
- 2 tbsp of virgin olive oil

- .25 c of lime juice
- .25 c of fresh cilantro leaves
- 1 avocado, ripe, pitted, chopped
- .5 c of red onion, sliced

First, separate your onion and set it aside in a bowl.

Combine avocado, cilantro, lime juice, garlic and salt in a bowl, then funnel into a food processor.

Process until a creamy consistency, make sure to get the bits on the side of the processor.

Before serving, take your green, beans, tomatoes, and corn, and toss them together in a large bowl. Add onions, apply the avocado dressing.

Toss salad and serve!

Creamy Cod and Tomato Sauce

The serving size for this meal is a quarter pound of cod and there are 4 servings prepared by this recipe. It will take you just under an hour to cook.

What's in it:

521 milligrams of potassium; 494 milligrams of sodium; 1 milligram of iron; 61 milligrams of calcium; 14 milligrams of vitamin C; 721 milligrams of vitamin A; 0 grams of added sugars; 3 grams of sugar; 74 milligrams of cholesterol; 19 grams of protein; 6 grams of carbs; 2 grams of fiber; 10 grams of fat; a total of 219 Calories

Ingredients:

- .5 tsp of cornstarch
- .25 c of half-and-half or heavy cream
- 1 14-oz can of tomatoes, diced
- .75 c of white wine
- 2 minced garlic cloves
- 1 chopped shallot
- 1 tbsp of extra-virgin olive oil

- .25 tsp of ground pepper, freshly ground
- .5 tsp of divided salt
- 3 tsp of fresh thyme, chopped and divided
- 1.25 lb. of cod or tilapia, cut into quarters

First, you want to pre-season your fish with a single tsp of thyme, plus .25 tsp of salt and pepper.

Next, you want to begin heating your olive oil in a skillet, medium setting. Add your minced garlic, shallot, and a tsp of thyme. Cook that for one minute, stirring until softened.

Add your wine, tomatoes, and fish to the pan, allowing it to simmer. You're going to want to cover the fish and let it cook, for about 4 to 6 minutes.

Move your fish over to a large plate, keep it warm.

Whisk your cornstarch and cream together into a bowl of suitable size. Now toss this into the pan with the remaining seasonings! Let it all blend and cook for approximately one to two minutes.

Serve fish and sauce!

Chicken Wrap with Curry Apples

This recipe will prepare two servings, with a single serving being one wrap. It should take you about 40 minutes to make in total.

What's in it:

260 milligrams of potassium; 363 milligrams of sodium; 2 milligrams of iron; 74 milligrams of calcium; 1 milligram of vitamin C; 181 milligrams of vitamin A; 4 grams of sugar; 65 milligrams of cholesterol; 28 grams of protein; 17 grams of carbs; 8 grams of fiber; 10 grams of fat; a total of 244 Calories

Ingredients:

- 12 spinach leaves or 2 large lettuce leaves
- 2 warmed 7-inch flour tortillas
- .25 tsp of curry
- 12 tbsp of Greek yogurt, plain
- 2 tbsp of light mayo
- 2 tbsp of red onions, chopped
- .5 c of green apple, chopped

- 1 c of shredded chicken breast, cooked

First, grab a medium bowl. You're going to toss your apples, mayo, Greek yogurt, curry, chicken and red onions in. Shake it up.

Line the tortilla wraps with the spinach or lettuce leaf of your choice. Apply your wrap mix generously, then roll your tortillas up!

Done!

Broccoli, Ginger, and Roasted Salmon

The serving size for this meal is 4 ounces of salmon and 1.5 c of broccoli, the recipe will prepare 4 servings. It will take you approximately 50 minutes in total.

What's in it:

1,044 milligrams of potassium; 603 milligrams of sodium; 3 milligrams of iron; 158 milligrams of calcium; 106 milligrams of vitamin C; 2,205 milligrams of vitamin A; 7 grams of added sugars; 10 grams of sugar; 66 milligrams of cholesterol; 34 grams of protein; 17 grams of carbs; 2 grams of fiber; 13 grams of fat; a total of 323 Calories

Ingredients:

- 2 tsp of sesame seeds, toasted
- 1.25 lb. of salmon, severed into four portions
- 1 tbsp of molasses
- 8 c of broccoli florets, large, with stalks attached
- .25 tsp of divided salt

- 1 tbsp of fresh ginger, grated
- 1.5 tbsp of rice vinegar
- 1.5 tbsp of tamari
- 1.5 tbsp of dark sesame oil

First, get your over ready. It should be preheated to about 425 degrees. Your baking sheet will need to be coated as well.

Combine your ginger, tamari, vinegar, oil, and .125 tsp of salt into a bowl. Whisk thoroughly. Add your broccoli florets in, giving them a good toss. You want them to be soaked.

Transfer the broccoli into the pan but allow the marinade to remain in the bowl. Now take your molasses and whisk it into the bowl with the marinade.

Time to get your broccoli crispy. Throw them in the oven for about five minutes, then slide them to the side and place your salmon beside it. Season your salmon well with the remaining salt and the glaze from your bowl.

Roast your salmon until it is fully cooked through. Should be about 7 to 10 minutes.

Decorate with your toasted sesame seeds.

Done!

Saag Made Simple

One serving of this recipe is a single cup, and there are about 4 servings in total. Preparation time will be 50 minutes.

What's in it:

815 milligrams of potassium; 641 milligrams of sodium; 3 milligrams of iron; 700 milligrams of calcium; 10 milligrams of vitamin C; 0 grams of added sugars; 11 grams of sugar; 64 grams of cholesterol; 25 grams of protein; 19 grams of carbs; 5 grams of fiber; 24 grams of fat; 382 Calories

Ingredients:

- Plain yogurt, 2 c
- 20 oz of frozen spinach, chopped
- 1 tsp of cumin, ground
- 2 tsp of masala
- 1 tbsp of fresh ginger, minced
- 1 minced clove of garlic
- 1 chopped jalapeno pepper
- 1 finely chopped onion

- 2 tbsp of olive oil
- .25 tsp of turmeric, ground
- 8 oz of paneer cheese cubes

Add paneer to a bowl and toss it with turmeric. Added a single tbsp of heated oil to a skill, place over medium heat. Toss in your paneer and cook it well, flipping until browned on both sides. Move to a plate.

Now you want to take your remaining oil and add it to a pan. Throw in your chopped and minced bits, the onion, and jalapeno, stirring until they're cooked to a golden brown.

Combine with garm masala, cumin, garlic, and ginger. Stir and cook until seasoning is evenly distributed. Mix in spinach and salt.

Cook for about 3 minutes, then take it off the heat. Add your yogurt and paneer, mixing thoroughly.

Done!

Oats with Bananas and Blueberries

This recipe will prepare one serving, which is 1.5 c of oats. It will take you 10 minutes to prepare but will be left sitting overnight. This is a meal for the next day.

What's in it:

452 milligrams of potassium; 147 milligrams of sodium; 2 milligrams of iron; 84 milligrams of calcium; 12 milligrams of vitamin C; 328 milligrams of vitamin A; 4 grams of added sugar; 20 grams of sugar; 6 grams of protein; 57 grams of carbs; 7 grams of fiber; 6 grams of fat; 285 Calories in total

Ingredients:

- 1 tbsp of flaked coconut
- .5 c of fresh blueberries
- A pinch of salt
- 1 tsp of maple syrup
- .5 banana, mashed
- .5 tbsp of chia seeds

- .5 cup of oats
- .5 cup of coconut milk

This is probably the easiest recipe in the world, with the longest wait time. Grab your coconut milk and pour it into a single pt. jar. Add your salt, maple syrup, banana, chia seeds, and oats. Shake well. Place coconut flakes and blueberries on top, reseal. Let sit in the refrigerator until the next morning.

Mixed Greens and Winter Squash, with Roasted Chicken

One serving of this meal is 2 c salad, 3 oz chicken and 2 slices of squash. The recipe will prepare four servings and will take you one hour and twenty minutes to make.

What's in it:

10 grams of sugars; 84 grams of cholesterol; 31 grams of protein; 39 grams of carbs; 7 grams of fiber; 17 grams of fat; 415 Calories

Ingredients:

- 4 tsp of roasted pumpkin seeds
- 4 tsp of parmesan cheese, grated
- 8 c of mixed greens
- 1.5 tsp of thyme leaves, fresh
- 1 tbsp of maple syrup, pure
- 1 lb. of chicken breast, boneless
- .5 tsp of salt
- 1 tsp of pepper, ground

- 2 tbsp of lemon juice
- 1 tsp of lemon zest, grated
- 1 tbsp of fresh or dried rosemary
- 3 minced garlic cloves
- 2 tbsp of mustard grain
- 3 tbsp of olive oil
- 2.5 lbs. acorn squash

You'll want to begin with preheating your over to 425 degrees Fahrenheit. Coat a cooking sheet, preferably large, with cooking spray.

Now take your squash, rinse it, and cut it in half across the length. Remove all seeds, then cut into inch wide slices.

Take .25 tsp of salt, .5 tsp of pepper, .5 tbsp of lemon juice, your lemon zest, and 1.5 tbsp of garlic, rosemary, and mustard, and 1 tbsp of oil. Mixed them all together in a bowl, then toss your chicken and squash in.

Place as a single layer on the pan you coated earlier.

Bake well, for at least 20 – 22 minutes, until the squash browns and chicken are cooked through.

Place chicken on cutting board and slice it up.

Whisk your remaining oil, lemon juice, maple syrup, thyme, pepper, and salt into a bowl, and add your greens. Mix again, to make sure to get green fully coated.

Serve greens first, then chicken and squash. Top with parmesan and pumpkin seed.

Done!

Falafel with Tahini Sauce

The traditional serving size for this meal is 3 falafel cakes. The recipe will prepare 4 servings. It will take you about an hour to prepare.

What's in it:

6 grams of sugar; 11 grams of protein; 34 grams of carbs; 7 grams of fiber; 17 grams of fat; 331 Calories in total

Ingredients:

- .25 tsp of baking soda
- .5 tsp of salt
- 1 tbsp of cumin
- 1 tbsp of lemon juice
- 4 tbsp of olive oil
- 2 cloves of garlic
- .25 c of onion, chopped
- .5 c of parsley packed down
- 1 c of dried chickpeas, soaked
- Ingredients for Sauce:
- Lemon zest

- .25 tsp of salt
- 1 clove of grated garlic
- 1 tbsp of olive oil
- 2 tbsp of lemon juice
- 3 tbsp of warm water
- 3 tbsp of tahini

After your chickpeas have been soaked, you are going to drain them and toss them into the food processor. The baking soda, salt, cumin, lemon juice, onion, garlic, parsley, and a single tbsp of oil will join the chickpeas in the processor. Add water if it is necessary. You'll want this mix to hold together on its own.

Take 3 tbsp of mix, shape into a patty. You should be able to craft about twelve of them.

Heat 2 tbsp of olive oil in a large skillet, making sure heat is at a medium to high range. Once olive oil is spread evenly, lower the heat to medium. Cook patties until a deep brown, almost golden, color on the bottom. Flip the patties, adding the remaining olive oil, and cook two to four minutes more.

Now to prepare your sauce. Simply combine tahini, water, garlic, oil, salt, and lemon juice into a bowl, and stir thoroughly. Add lemon zest, then stick it in the fridge!

Shepherd's Pie, Vegan

This recipe will prepare 6 servings and take a total of one hour to prepare.

What's in it:

1317 milligrams of sodium; 20 grams of protein; 64 grams of carbs; 24 grams of fat; 552 Calories

Ingredients:

- .5 c of imitation cheddar cheese, soy cheese
- 14 oz of ground beef substitute
- 1 pinch of black pepper, ground
- 1 minced garlic clove
- 1 tsp of Italian seasoning
- 1 chopped tomato
- .5 c of frozen peas
- 3 chopped celery stalks
- 2 chopped carrots
- 1 chopped yellow onion
- 1 tbsp of vegetable oil
- 2 tsp of salt
- 3 tbsp of cream cheese, vegan substitute

- .25 c of olive oil
- .5 cup of soy milk
- .5 cup of mayo, vegan
- 5 peeled and cubed russet potatoes

First, you're going to want to boil your potatoes. Place them over medium heat in a pot, and allow to boil until tender, then drain. Mash the potatoes, stirring in your salt, vegan cheese, olive oil, vegan mayo, and soy milk. Mix until creamy and place to the side, covered.

Now, preheat your oven. 400 degrees should be more than high enough. You'll need a deep baking dish to cook within, spray it down with cooking oil.

Cook your vegetable oil in a skill, adding the tomato, frozen peas, celery, carrots, and onion so that they get nice and tender. Season with your pepper, garlic, and Italian seasonings.

Lower the heat of the skillet and add your vegan ground beef mixture over the veggies. Cook until the mixture is visibly hot, then add it to the bottom of the baking dish.

Place the mashed potato on top. Spread shredded soy cheese over potatoes.

Bake in the oven for 20 minutes, or until the cheeses are melted and browned.

Chickpeas, Spinach, and Eggs in Sauce

The serving size for this meal is one egg with .75 c of sauce. It prepares four servings and will take 45 minutes to cook.

What's in it:

6 g sugar; 203 milligrams of cholesterol; 14 grams of protein; 26 grams of carbs; 6 grams of fiber; 18 grams of fat; 323 Calories

Ingredients:

- .5 tsp of pepper
- 1 tbsp of fresh thyme, chopped
- 4 eggs
- .5 tsp of salt
- .25 c of heavy cream
- 1 can of chickpeas, make sure to rinse
- 2 c of crushed tomatoes
- 4 sliced garlic cloves
- 4 c of chopped baby spinach

- 2 tbsp of olive oil

Begin by preparing a skillet over heat, spreading the oil across the surface evenly. Now toss your garlic and spinach in, allowing it to cook for about two minutes. Garlic should be browned, and the spinach should be wilted.

Lower the heat to medium. Gather your salt, cream, tomatoes, and chickpeas. Add them to your skillet. Maintain a simmer, adjusting the heat accordingly.

Crack your egg into a bowl, but do not break the yolk. In your skillet, create a well to pour the egg into. Pour egg in, do not break the yolk. You want your egg whites to be mostly contained within the sauce.

Repeat this process with the other eggs, creating wells and pouring the egg in without breaking.

Sprinkle your thyme across the top of the meal, and cover for about six to eight minutes, or until the eggs are cooked through. Take the skillet off the heat, garnish with pepper.

Done!

Baked Peppers Stuffed with Eggs

Serving size for this dish is one bell pepper with egg, this recipe prepares six servings. It will take about one hour to make.

Ingredients:

- Fresh black pepper
- 2 c marinara sauce
- 6 eggs
- .25 c of crumbled feta
- .5 c of ricotta cheese
- .25 c of brandy
- Kosher salt
- 1 tsp of dried thyme
- 1 lb. of diced squash, peeled and seeded
- .5 c of chopped onion
- 2 cloves of diced garlic
- 1 tbsp of olive oil
- 2 tbsp of butter
- 3 bell peppers

Begin by heating your oven to 400 degrees. Half your peppers, emptying them of seeds and ribs. Place to the side in a bowl or dish. Add .25 c of water to the bowl. Sprinkle with pepper and salt, and cover with plastic. Microwave for 5 minutes.

Next, you are going to add your butter and oil to a skillet. Once the oil is heated, toss in the garlic and let it cook for a minute, then add the onion. Let onion sauté. Combine squash, thyme, and salt, then add it to the skillet. Cook for another 5 minutes. Take the skillet off the heat and add your brandy. Mix, and then place the skillet back onto the stove. Once squash is softened, you can add the cheese and cover, allowing the cheese to melt.

Next, line the bottom of your baking dish with marinara. Place the peppers on the pan, with the cup side facing up. Fill them with your squash mix, leaving enough room for the egg. Bake your peppers in the oven for 10 minutes.

Once baking is down, crack an egg into a measuring cup, careful not to break the yolk. Pour into the peppers, but do not let them overflow.

Season with black pepper, then bake for another 10-12 minutes. Once eggs have baked to a white, and are settled in peppers, remove from oven and serve. Add extra marinara and feta if desired.

Tofurrito, Vegan Breakfast Wrap

The serving size for this meal is one wrap, and the recipe itself makes four burritos.

What's in it:

16 grams of Proteins; 3 grams of sugar; 8 grams of fiber; 53 grams of carbs; 772 milligrams of sodium; 19 grams of fat; 441 Calories in total

Ingredients for the tofu:

- .25 c of parsley, minced
- A dash of cayenne pepper
- .25 teaspoon of sea salt
- 1 teaspoon of yeast
- .5 teaspoon of cumin
- .5 teaspoon of chili powder
- 1 tablespoon of hummus
- 3 cloves of garlic
- 1 tsp of oil
- 12 oz package of firm tofu
- Ingredients for vegetables:
- 2 cups chopped kale

- .5 teaspoons of chili powder
- .5 teaspoon of ground cumin
- 1 dash of salt
- 1 teaspoon of oil
- 1 bell pepper, sliced thin
- 5 baby potatoes, chopped
- Other Ingredients:
- Chunky salsa, or hot sauce
- Cilantro
- 1 avocado, ripe
- 3-4 large flour tortillas

Like most recipes, we begin by heating our oven. Raise the temperature to 400 degrees Fahrenheit. Line your baking sheet with parchment paper. Wrap your tofu in a clean towel and pan on top. This is to press out extra moisture. Once this is done, crumble it with a fork and put it to the side.

On your baking sheet, layer your potatoes and red peppers, coating them with oil and spice. Mix them, bake them for 15 minutes or so. Once they are golden brown, you're going to toss some kale in and mix it with the peppers and potatoes. Let that bake until wilted.

While this is happening, take your skill and heat it up. Medium heat should do the trick. Add your oil and tofu, cooking it up until browned.

Now, take your bowl, and combine hummus, cumin, yeast, salt, cayenne, and chili powder. Stir those together, then add water until a sauce is formed. Once thickened, add in your parsley and mix some more. Take this sauce, pour it into the skillet, and cook your tofu for another 3-5 minutes.

Now, take your tortilla wraps and lay them out, doling out your tofu and veggies in generous proportions. It will take some effort to wrap them up, so make sure to tuck!

Noodle Bowl with Beef

This recipe will prepare four servings and take you an hour and a half.

What's in it:

4 grams of added sugars; 9 grams of sugar; 55 milligrams of cholesterol; 24 grams of protein; 30 grams of carbs; 3 grams of fiber; 14 grams of fat; 348 Calories

Ingredients:

- Lime slices
- 2 tbsp of fresh basil, minced
- .5 c of baby carrots
- 1 c of red cabbage, shredded
- 1 c of cucumber, chopped
- 12 oz beef steak, cut into bite-sized strips
- Cooking spray
- .125 tsp of red pepper
- .25 tsp of salt
- 2 minced cloves of garlic
- 1 tbsp of fresh ginger, grated

- 1 tbsp of honey
- 1 tbsp of canola oil
- 1 tbsp of sesame oil
- 1.5 tbsp of lime juice
- 2 tbsp of soy sauce
- 2 tbsp of rice vinegar
- 4 oz of rice noodles or spaghetti

Take the pasta from the package and cook it, approximately 5 to 10 minutes. Once drained, store in a pan with a cover, as you will want to keep it warm.

In a bowl suitable for mixing, whisk together all ingredients from rice vinegar to red pepper. Stop at cooking spray.

With your cooking spray, coat a skillet and heat it. Your heat should be set somewhere between medium and high. Begin cooking your meat, half the portion at a time, until browned. Store it somewhere to be kept warm.

Lower your heat. From the sauce bowl earlier, pour .25 c into the skillet and cook it until evaporated. You want the brown flakes, don't worry. Now add your meat, with the juices, back to the skillet, and cook for another couple of minutes.

Separate pasta, pouring the sauce over it generously. Take your cucumbers, cabbage, and carrots, toss them on top. Finally, add meat, garnish with basil, and pour more sauce if desired. Serve with limes.

Vegetable Stir-fry

The serving size for this is one plate of stir fry, and the recipe makes four servings. It will take you one hour to prepare this dish.

What's in it:

7 grams of carbs; 5 grams of sugar; 1.7 grams of fiber; 122 Calories

Ingredients:

- 2 tablespoons of fresh herbs, cilantro, and basil, chopped
- 1 tablespoon of garlic, ginger, and shallots
- 2 pounds of veggies, cut into bite-sized pieces.
- 1 pound of protein, chicken or beef, cut into bite-sized pieces

Grab your wok, we're making stir fry. Place it over medium heat and allow it to get extremely hot. Add two tbsp of oil, coat the pan.

Add meat and cook until browned all around, making sure it is cooked through and sizzling. Remove and place on a plate.

Add your thick veggies, like peppers or carrots, into the pan. Cook them up for about a minute, then add any other vegetables.

Now toss in your garlic, ginger, and shallots, with some additional oil. Keep them stirred to avoid burning.

Return your meat to the wok, along with a sauce of your choice, and cook until the whole thing is bubbling.

Remove from heat and serve! This dish goes great with brown rice.

Essential Chopped Salad

2 c of salad will fill you up, and this recipe will make four servings. It takes approximately fifty minutes to prepare.

What's in it:

11 grams of sugar; 7 milligrams of cholesterol; 9 grams of protein; 39 grams of carbs; 7 grams of fiber; 23 grams of fat; a total of 376 Calories

Ingredients:

- Seasonings: Tsp of salt and pepper
- 1 peeled clove of garlic
- 1 tbsp of lemon juice
- .25 c of mayo
- .25 cup of buttermilk
- .5 c of fresh basil, chopped
- .25 cup of currants
- .25 cup of pepitas, toasted
- 1 ripe avocado
- 1 c of cherry tomatoes, cut in half
- 1 c of corn kernels

- 6 c of baby arugula
- .5 cup of couscous
- .75 c of water

Start by boiling your water in a saucepan. Once this is done, you'll add your couscous, letting it lower to a simmer. Cook this for 8 to 10 minutes. Store couscous in a mesh sleeve and rinse with water.

On a serving platter, garnish freely with arugula. Apply avocado, tomatoes, corn, currants, pepitas, and couscous in lines over arugula.

In a blender, combine your salt, pepper, garlic, lemon juice, mayo, buttermilk, and basil. Use pulse setting, and ensure it comes out smooth.

Pour over salad and enjoy.

Coleslaw with Chicken and Pineapple

One serving is half a chicken breast and 1.5 c of slaw. This recipe will prepare four servings in 50 minutes.

What's in it:

13 grams of sugar; 27 grams of protein; 19 grams of carbs; 3 grams of fiber; 7 grams of fat; 238 Calories

Ingredients:

- 4 Boneless chicken breasts, cut into half
- 2 tsp of jerk seasoning
- 2 tsp of flour
- 4 tsp of brown sugar
- 2 tbsp of cider vinegar
- Half a pineapple
- 2 c of red cabbage, shredded
- 3 heads of baby bok choy, thin slices

In a large bowl, you are going to prepare the coleslaw. Take 2 tsp of brown sugar and apple cider vinegar and add them to the bowl. Toss in pineapple, cabbage, and bok choy.

In a plastic bag, such as a refrigerator or freezer bag, combine flour, jerk seasoning, and 2 tsp of brown sugar. Throw in the chicken and shake it.

Now, on a skillet, cook your chicken until it is no longer raw. Turn once about 6 minutes in to cook the other side.

Once cooked, take the chicken and place it on a cutting board. Slide and combine with slaw.

Shrimp, Edamame, and Slaw

This recipe will prepare four servings in thirty minutes.

What's in it:

3 grams of sugar; 137 milligrams of cholesterol; 28 grams of protein; 20 grams of carbs; 9 grams of fiber; 19 grams of fat; and 364 Calories

Ingredients:

- 12 oz peeled and cooked shrimp
- Half a lime, juiced
- 1 avocado, diced
- 2 c of frozen edamame, thawed
- 1 recipe of slaw, such as the one above

First, you will need to have some coleslaw prepared. If you don't have a recipe already, you can use the one above. Now add edamame into this slaw and put it to the side.

Combine lime juice and avocado in a bull, mixing.

Top the slaw with the shrimp, avocado, and then separate into containers to be refrigerated. Recipes like these are a "take it to work" meal.

Bananas and Peanut Butter on Toast

This recipe will prepare one portion in 10 minutes.

What's in it:

14 grams of sugar; 8 grams of protein; 38 grams of carbs; 5 grams of fiber; 9 grams of fat; 266 Calories

Ingredients:

- A dash of cinnamon
- 1 banana, sliced
- A tbsp of peanut butter
- 1 slice of toast, whole wheat or otherwise

This is a quick and satisfying recipe that anyone can make in under ten minutes.

Simply toast bread to your preference and slice your banana in the meantime.

Once toasted, spread peanut butter over toast.

Place banana slices on top of the peanut butter, and sprinkle with cinnamon. Great to bring to work with you, if you aren't eating in the morning.

A Medley of Chickpeas, Green and Roasted Salmon

This recipe prepares four servings and is completed in a little over an hour and a half.

What's in it:

37 grams of protein; 23 grams of carbs; 2 grams of sugar; 6 grams of fiber; 22 grams of fat

Ingredients:

- 1.5 pounds of salmon, split up into portions
- .25 c of water
- 10 c of kale, chopped
- .25 tsp of garlic powder
- .5 tsp of pepper, ground
- .24 c of chives and dill
- .25 cup of mayo
- .75 c of buttermilk
- 1 can of rinsed chickpeas
- .5 tsp of salt
- 1 tbsp of paprika

- 2 tbsp of olive oil

Place your pan on the middle rack in an oven preheated to 425 degrees.

Mix one tbsp of oil, paprika, and .25 tsp of salt into a bowl. Dry your chickpeas off, then add it to your mixture. Spread this over the baking sheet. Bake them on the highest rack, for thirty minutes.

Take your buttermilk, herbs, .25 tsp of pepper and garlic, mayo, and blend them until smooth.

Heat your oil in a skillet. Toss kale and cook until wilted. Add water and cook kale until soft. Remove from heat, stir in some salt.

Chickpeas should be done by now, so pull them out of the oven and line the side of the pan with them, making room for your salmon. Season with remaining seasoning and bake anywhere from 5 minutes to 8 minutes.

Take your dressing from earlier apply to the salmon. Serve with your chickpea and kale side.

Single Pan Veggie and Chicken

This recipe will take twenty minutes to cook and yield two servings.

What's in it:

42 grams of protein; 10 grams of carbs; 5 grams of sugar; 241 Calories

Ingredients:

- .25 tsp paprika
- 1 tsp of Italian seasonings
- .5 tsp of black pepper
- .5 tsp of salt
- 2 tbsp of olive oil
- .5 c of tomatoes
- 1 c of broccoli florets
- 1 zucchini chopped
- .5 onion chopped
- 1 c bell pepper chopped
- 2 chicken breasts chopped

Set your over to 500 degrees.

Take your veggies and rinse them. Once clean, chop your veggies and blend them in a mixing bowl. On another platter, chop up your chicken into cubes.

Mix the veggies and chicken into one pan, with olive oil and seasonings.

Bake for as long as needed, until veggies are charred, and chicken is browned.

Salmon in a Jiff, Maple Style

This recipe will make four servings and takes about 10 minutes to prepare.

What's in it:

20 grams of sugar; 138 milligrams of sodium; 50 grams of protein; 28 grams of fat; 468 Calories

Ingredients:

- 3 tbsp of pure maple syrup
- 1.5 lbs. of salmon fillet
- .5 tsp of salt
- 2 tsp of brown sugar
- 1 tbsp of paprika
- 1 tbsp of chili powder

First, set your oven to broil. Take a medium sized pan, line it with aluminum foil, then apply an ample coating of cooking spray.

With a bowl near, mix your seasonings together. This includes salt, sugar, paprika, and chili powder.

Apply this mix over the salmon in a fine dusting.

Line the baking sheet with salmon fillets, and broil for 10 minutes. This time may change depending on the size of salmon.

Once baked for 10 minutes, remove the salmon from oven and give it a rub of pure maple syrup. This will meld with the spices baked in and give an amazing flavor.

Immediately place back in over, and broil for a couple more minutes. Remove from oven and serve.

Spaghetti Heaven, Mediterranean Veggies and Chicken

This meal can be prepared in 30 minutes and will provide 4 servings.

What's in it:

532 Calories; 6 grams of sugar; 21 grams of protein; 27 grams of fat

Ingredients:

3 tbs of olive oil

8 ounces of pasta

3 cloves of garlic

8 ounces of fresh spinach

.25 c of basil

Roma tomatoes, 4, chopped

.25 tsp of salt

.25 tsp of pepper flakes

.5 lb. chicken breast

.25 c of sun-dried tomatoes

First, you're going to want to cook up the sun-dried tomatoes. Add them, and two tbsp of olive oil to a skillet on medium heat.

Next, cook your chicken up right beside it! Season with red pepper and salt. Cook your chicken until there is no trace of pink anymore.

Add your Roma tomatoes, chopped up, some basil leaves, garlic, and the spinach into your skillet. Cook this for about five minutes, watching for the wilting signs of the spinach. Pull it off the heat.

Cook your pasta, making sure it gets no further than al dente. Drain it and toss it into the skillet with veggies and chicken.

Now reheat it in the skillet and toss the rest of your seasoning it.

Add more olive oil, if desired.

Serve and enjoy!

Avocado, Chickpeas, and Cranberries Salad Sandwich

This recipe only takes 10 minutes to prepare and will provide two servings.

What's in it:

12.3 grams of protein; 17.3 grams of fiber; 10.7 grams of sugars; 60.5 grams of carbs; 15.3 grams of fat; 406 Calories

Ingredients:

- Salt and pepper for taste
- .25 c of cranberries
- 2 tsp of freshly squeezed lemons
- 1 ripened avocado
- 15 oz of rinsed chickpeas

Another quick "bring it to work" meal. Take your chickpeas, drain them and rinse them. In a bowl, you will smash them up, then mix in your avocado. Smash this as well, blending into a chunky paste. Add lemon juice, cranberries and season with your chosen blend. Salt and pepper added in last.

Keep this in the fridge until serving.

When you're ready to make lunch, just toast up your bread and spread this on. Garnish with onions, spinach, and arugula for some snap!

Pasta Salad, Tahini Style

This recipe will serve 4 to 6 people and will take a total of 40 minutes to prepare.

Ingredients:

- Sea salt and ground pepper
- .25 c of pine nuts
- 8 basil leaves, sliced thin
- 4 oil rich sun-dried tomatoes
- 1 cup sliced cherry tomatoes
- 1 small zucchini, sliced
- 2 c pasta
- 1 c green beans
- 3 c broccoli florets
- Ingredients for Tahini:
- Tbsp of water
- .5 tsp of salt
- .5 tsp of maple syrup
- .5 tsp of Dijon mustard
- 1 clove of garlic, diced
- 2 tbsp of white wine vinegar
- 3 tbsp of fresh lemon juice

- 3 tbsp of tahini
- 3 tbsp of olive oil

Grab yourself a bowl, and throw in the olive oil, tahini, vinegar, lemon, salt, water, garlic, mustard, and maple syrup. Blend it up.

Now, bring a pot of water to boil. Once boiling, cook up broccoli and green beans until tender, but still green. Remove from water, submerge in ice water prepared ahead of time. This will keep it from cooking further. Once veggies are cool, drain water and store veggies on a towel to dry.

In another pot, boil more water. Cook your pasta until it is at al dente level. Drain and run cold water over it.

Now, combine the remainder of your ingredients into a bowl! Drizzle with the dressing and toss. Store into a container to take with you to work. Don't forget to garnish with the pine nuts.

Top Tier Turkey Lettuce Wraps

This recipe can be prepared in thirty minutes and will yield six servings.

What's in it:

3.4 grams of sugar; 23 grams of protein; 1 gram of fiber; 8 grams of carbs; 4.3 grams of fat; 162 Calories in total

Ingredients:

- 12 lettuce leaves
- A dash of salt
- 2 teaspoons of roasted chili paste
- 1 tablespoon of rice vinegar
- 2 tablespoons of soy sauce, low sodium
- 3 tablespoons of hoisin sauce
- 8 oz can of water chestnuts, chopped
- 4 green onions, sliced thin
- .125 teaspoon of ground ginger
- 1 minced garlic clove
- 1 tablespoon of olive oil

- 1.25 lb. of ground turkey, lean

Begin with heating your skillet, applying your tbsp of oil to the pan. Once well coated, you can begin cooking up your garlic and ginger, set the flavor. Once the garlic is slightly browned, toss in turkey meat, stirring it until it is falling apart.

Combine onions, water chestnuts, and your cooked turkey meat into a bowl, and stir it up.

In a separate bowl, mix your sauce. Add red chili paste, hoisin, rice vinegar, and soy sauce. Once blended together, pour over turkey mix.

Spread your lettuce leaf out, add mix, wrap and enjoy!

Conclusion

Thank you for making it through to the end of *Intermittent Fasting: The Code of Weight Loss Mastery in 2019 for Beginner and Advanced. Eat and Stop Obesity.* Let's hope it was informative and able to provide you with all the tools you need to achieve your goals whatever they may be. We've covered the history of Intermittent Fasting and provided every piece of potential data to support what you have heard. You now know about several ways you can begin losing weight, without all the pesky traps in dieting. Not only that, you know that fasting won't just shed those pounds, but it will extend years on your life and make you an overall healthier person. Hopefully, you're as excited to fast as all the wise men and women of our history who have used it before you. Now that you understand exactly how to fast, and what will happen once you do, the path ahead is clear.

The next step is to begin your Intermittent Fasting journey! There are more resources out there, but if you are truly satisfied with this book you can always start fasting today. If you have any questions, flip back a few pages and reread! If the answers aren't there, which they should be, then feel free to do more research. Remember, it's your body. Intermittent Fasting is just the best way to preserve it.

Finally, if you found this book useful in any way, a review on Amazon is always appreciated!

Made in the USA
San Bernardino, CA
18 November 2019